Caries Management

Editors

SANDRA GUZMÁN-ARMSTRONG
MARGHERITA FONTANA
MARCELLE M. NASCIMENTO
ANDREA G. FERREIRA ZANDONA

DENTAL CLINICS OF NORTH AMERICA

www.dental.theclinics.com

October 2019 • Volume 63 • Number 4

ELSEVIER

1600 John F. Kennedy Boulevard • Suite 1800 • Philadelphia, Pennsylvania, 19103-2899

http://www.dental.theclinics.com

DENTAL CLINICS OF NORTH AMERICA Volume 63, Number 4
October 2019 ISSN 0011-8532, ISBN: 978-0-323-67337-2

Editor: John Vassallo; j.vassallo@elsevier.com
Developmental Editor: Laura Fisher

Dental Clinics of North America (ISSN 0011-8532) is published quarterly by Elsevier Inc., 360 Park Avenue South, New York, NY 10010-1710. Months of issue are January, April, July, and October. Business and Editorial Offices: 1600 John F. Kennedy Boulevard, Suite 1800, Philadelphia, PA 19103-2899. Periodicals postage paid at New York, NY and additional mailing offices. Subscription prices are $304.00 per year (domestic individuals), $603.00 per year (domestic institutions), $100.00 per year (domestic students/residents), $366.00 per year (Canadian individuals), $782.00 per year (Canadian institutions), $424.00 per year (international individuals), $782.00 per year (international institutions), and $200.00 per year (international and Canadian students/residents). International air speed delivery is included in all *Clinics* subscription prices. All prices are subject to change without notice. **POSTMASTER:** Send address changes to *Dental Clinics of North America*, Elsevier Health Sciences Division, Subscription Customer Service, 3251 Riverport Lane, Maryland Heights, MO 63043. **Customer Service (orders, claims, online, change of address): Elsevier Health Sciences Division, Subscription Customer Service, 3251 Riverport Lane, Maryland Heights, MO 63043. Tel: 1-800-654-2452 (U.S. and Canada). Fax: 314-447-8029. E-mail: journalscustomer service-usa@elsevier.com (for print support); journalsonlinesupport-usa@elsevier.com (for online support).**

Reprints. For copies of 100 or more, of articles in this publication, please contact the Commercial Reprints Department, Elsevier Inc., 360 Park Avenue South, New York, NY 10010-1710. Tel.: 212-633-3874; Fax: 212-633-3820; E-mail: reprints@elsevier.com.

The *Dental Clinics of North America* is covered in *MEDLINE/PubMed (Index Medicus), Current Contents/Clinical Medicine, ISI/BIOMED* and *Clinahl.*

Contributors

EDITORS

SANDRA GUZMÁN-ARMSTRONG, DDS, MS
Clinical Professor and Advanced Education Program Co-Director, Department of Operative Dentistry, The University of Iowa College of Dentistry and Dental Clinics, Iowa City, Iowa, USA

MARGHERITA FONTANA, DDS, PhD
Clifford Nelson Endowed Professor of Dentistry, Cariology Discipline Co-coordinator, Department of Cariology, Restorative Sciences and Endodontics, University of Michigan School of Dentistry, Ann Arbor, Michigan, USA

MARCELLE M. NASCIMENTO, DDS, MS, PhD
Associate Professor, Department of Restorative Dental Sciences, Division of Operative Dentistry, College of Dentistry, University of Florida, Gainesville, Florida, USA

ANDREA G. FERREIRA ZANDONA, DDS, MSD, PhD
Professor and Chair, Department of Comprehensive Care, Tufts University School of Dental Medicine, Tufts University, Boston, Massachusetts, USA

AUTHORS

FREDERICK EICHMILLER, DDS
Vice President and Science Officer, Delta Dental of Wisconsin, Stevens Point, Wisconsin, USA

RONALD ETTINGER, BDS, MDS, DDSc, DDSc(hc)
Professor Emeritus, Department of Prosthodontics, The University of Iowa College of Dentistry and Dental Clinics, Iowa City, Iowa, USA

ANDREA G. FERREIRA ZANDONA, DDS, MSD, PhD
Professor and Chair, Department of Comprehensive Care, Tufts University School of Dental Medicine, Tufts University, Boston, Massachusetts, USA

SUSAN A. FISHER-OWENS, MD, MPH, FAAP
Clinical Professor, Department of Pediatrics, School of Medicine, Clinical Professor, Department of Preventive and Restorative Dental Sciences, School of Dentistry, University of California, San Francisco, Zuckerberg San Francisco General Hospital, San Francisco, California, USA

KRISTEN FLICK, MSW
Social Worker, The University of Iowa College of Dentistry and Dental Clinics, Iowa City, Iowa, USA

MARGHERITA FONTANA, DDS, PhD
Clifford Nelson Endowed Professor of Dentistry, Cariology Discipline Co-coordinator, Department of Cariology, Restorative Sciences and Endodontics, University of Michigan School of Dentistry, Ann Arbor, Michigan, USA

SANDRA GUZMÁN-ARMSTRONG, DDS, MS
Clinical Professor and Advanced Education Program Co-Director, Department of Operative Dentistry, The University of Iowa College of Dentistry and Dental Clinics, Iowa City, Iowa, USA

JUDITH HABER, PhD, APRN, FAAN
Ursula Springer Leadership Professor in Nursing, Executive Director, Oral Health Nursing Education and Practice Program (OHNEP), NYU Rory Meyers College of Nursing, New York, New York, USA

ERIN HARTNETT, DNP, PPCNP-BC, CPNP
Director, Oral Health Nursing Education and Practice Program (OHNEP), NYU Rory Meyers College of Nursing, New York, New York, USA

JENNIFER HARTSHORN, DDS
Clinical Assistant Professor, Department of Preventive and Community Dentistry, The University of Iowa College of Dentistry and Dental Clinics, Iowa City, Iowa, USA

MARITA R. INGLEHART, Dipl. Psych., Dr. phil., Dr. phil. habil.
Professor of Dentistry, Department of Periodontics and Oral Medicine, School of Dentistry, Adjunct Professor, Department of Psychology, College of Literature, Science and Arts (LS&A), University of Michigan, Ann Arbor, Michigan, USA

DAVID C. JOHNSEN, DDS, MS
Professor and Dean, Department of Pediatric Dentistry, The University of Iowa College of Dentistry and Dental Clinics, Iowa City, Iowa, USA

MARTHA ANN KEELS, DDS, PhD
Adjunct Professor, Department of Pediatric Dentistry, University of North Carolina School of Dentistry, Adjunct Associate Professor, Department of Pediatrics, Duke University, Durham, North Carolina, USA

LEONARDO MARCHINI, DDS, MSD, PhD
Assistant Professor, Department of Preventive and Community Dentistry, The University of Iowa College of Dentistry and Dental Clinics, Iowa City, Iowa, USA

TERESA A. MARSHALL, PhD, RDN/LDN
Professor, Department of Preventive and Community Dentistry, The University of Iowa College of Dentistry and Dental Clinics, Iowa City, Iowa, USA

MARCELLE M. NASCIMENTO, DDS, MS, PhD
Associate Professor, Department of Restorative Dental Sciences, Division of Operative Dentistry, College of Dentistry, University of Florida, Gainesville, Florida, USA

FALK SCHWENDICKE, PhD, MDPH
Department for Operative and Preventive Dentistry, Charité – Universitätsmedizin Berlin, Berlin, Germany

ARZU TEZVERGIL-MUTLUAY, DDS, PhD
Professor, Department of Cariology and Restorative Dentistry, Adhesive Dentistry
Research Group, Institute of Dentistry, Turku University Hospital, TYKS, University of
Turku, Turku, Finland

LEO TJÄDERHANE, DDS, PhD
Professor, Department of Oral and Maxillofacial Diseases, University of Helsinki, Helsinki
University Hospital, Helsinki, Finland; Research Unit of Oral Health Sciences, Medical
Research Center Oulu (MRC Oulu), Oulu University Hospital, University of Oulu, Oulu,
Finland

Contents

Dental caries is closely related to a dysbiosis of the microbial consortia of supragingival oral biofilms driven by a sugar-frequent and acidic-pH environment. The pH is a key factor affecting the homeostasis of supragingival biofilms seen in health. There is increasing interest on the ecological dynamics of the oral microbiome and how a dysbiotic microbiota can be successfully replaced by health-beneficial flora. The concept of preventing the microbial dysbiosis related to caries through modulation of sugar intake and pH has fully emerged.

Acid produced during bacterial fermentation of carbohydrates dissolves tooth structure, leading to dental caries. Carbohydrates are a nutrient within foods, individual foods contain multitudinous differing nutrients in varying concentrations, and, ultimately, food choices and eating behaviors are associated with the caries process. Consideration of food choices and eating behaviors is necessary for effective caries prevention. This article (1) defines a healthy diet and eating behaviors as a foundation for caries prevention, (2) identifies food choices and eating behaviors associated with caries, (3) identifies diet-related screening and assessment tools for caries risk, and (4) provides counseling strategies to manage dental caries.

Dental caries and periodontal diseases are preventable. Nevertheless, they remain prevalent. Dental practices offer an ideal setting for educating patients about oral health-related behavior change. This article describes the motivational communication approach to changing behavior and applies it to a discussion of behavior change communication over the course of life. CONTENT considerations focus on identifying high-priority behaviors for change; patient affect, behavior, and cognition related to these behaviors, and understanding in which stage of change the patient is. Process the four principles of the Motivational Interviewing approach by Miller & Rollnick to analyze oral health-related behavior change over the life course.

oral health care. An increased awareness of these barriers, along with the resources that are available, may help dental providers to better reach their patients and manage dental caries.

The Interprofessional Role in Dental Caries Management: Ways Medical Providers Can Support Oral Health (Perspectives from a Physician)   669

Susan A. Fisher-Owens

Medical providers are important allies in the prevention of dental caries. Through raising the issue by asking about risks and strengths, offering anticipatory guidance and counseling, encouraging and following up on referrals, and applying preventive fluoride, medical providers can have a direct, positive impact on oral health. Further, improving communication with referrals, bidirectionally, benefits patient care as well as provider satisfaction. By collaborating on advocacy efforts, medical and dental providers can broaden their impact while building relationships, with the end goal of improved health for patients throughout their lifetime. Reintegrating the mouth into the body and oral health into systemic health has benefits for patients and providers alike, and can and should be accomplished in the medical home.

Caries Management Decision-Making: Diagnosis and Synthesis   679

Sandra Guzmán-Armstrong and David C. Johnsen

The purposes of this article are to (1) offer a critical thinking skill set in decision-making and synthesis for caries diagnosis, and risk-adjusted and personalized management based on emulating the intended activity of the expert, (2) offer patient/case scenarios for application of the critical thinking skill set, (3) compare and contrast the results of applying an algorithm and expert thought process approach to patient analyses, (4) offer characteristics of the person making decisions and synthesizing information, and (5) for patients with complex health and social histories, include perspectives from other health care team members.

Nonrestorative Management of Cavitated and Noncavitated Caries Lesions   695

Margherita Fontana

The objective of this article is to review evidence-based strategies available for the nonrestorative management of caries lesions, both cavitated and noncavitated. The goal is to help clinicians make appropriate decisions regarding nonrestorative management of caries lesions. In addition, in the decision-making process, clinicians must consider thresholds for restorative and nonrestorative care and strategies for nonrestorative management that are supported by best available evidence. It is important that this information be considered taking into account a provider's clinical expertise and a patient's treatment needs and preferences, in order to maintain health and preserve tooth structure.

Surgical Management of Caries Lesions: Selective Removal of Carious Tissues   705

Andrea G. Ferreira Zandona

Traditionally, before placing a restoration, excavation of tissues affected by caries was recommended. The goal was to have all walls of the cavity on sound, hard dentin, even when at risk of pulpal exposure. Current understanding of the caries process indicates that preserving tooth structure can lead to better long-term outcomes. Selective caries excavation refers to preserving tooth structure by delineating excavation in the pulpal and axial wall according to lesion severity and depth as well as pulpal health while keeping all cavity margins on sound tooth structure. Compounding evidence indicates that when a good marginal seal is present, the lesion will arrest.

Selective carious tissue-removal strategies require specific considerations in selection of restorative materials. A tight marginal seal placed over hard dentin and sound enamel is essential. For selective removal of carious tissue with permanent restoration, bioactive materials, such as high-viscosity glass-ionomer cement (HV-GIC) or calcium silicates, may be preferred over caries-affected firm or leathery dentin to improve remineralization. HV-GICs have the best clinical evidence of caries-arresting effect and demonstrate sufficient longevity as long-term provisional restorations that can later be used in open or closed sandwich restorations. As with any material, oral health maintenance remains important for long-term survival of restorations.

Caries management could provide a unique opportunity to model reform to the dental reimbursement system. To be successful we must first understand the scope and basis of many of the obstacles to reform. Reform must also provide value to all the players involved in benefit determination, provision of care, and payment for care. Value is viewed as outcomes achieved per dollar from the patient's perspective and over a complete cycle of care or management. Reimbursing for value requires measurement of value, and one hypothetical model for caries management is presented based on Michael Porter's hierarchy of outcome measures.

Caries is a chronic disease, with long-term sequelae, often initiated early in life. Managing caries and carious lesions often has long-term consequences. These consequences involve the health (or its absence) generated by a caries management strategy, but also costs. This article discusses the long-term health and costs consequences resulting from different caries management strategies. It is demonstrated why, and under which circumstances, minimal invasive caries management may be beneficial for patients, but also for health services, with regard to both health gained and costs generated. Moreover, possible factors influencing the cost-effectiveness of different caries management strategies will be discussed.

DENTAL CLINICS OF NORTH AMERICA

THE CLINICS ARE AVAILABLE ONLINE!
Access your subscription at:
www.theclinics.com

DENTAL CLINICS OF NORTH AMERICA

SERIES OF RELATED INTEREST

Atlas of the Oral and Maxillofacial Surgery Clinics
http://www.oralmaxsurgeryatlas.theclinics.com

Oral and Maxillofacial Surgery Clinics
http://www.oralmaxsurgery.theclinics.com

Preface
Dental Caries: Evidence and Interdisciplinary Person-Centered Care Considerations for Management Over Time

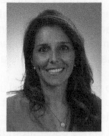

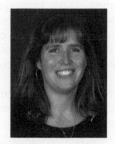

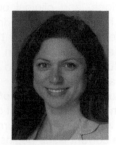

Sandra Guzmán-Armstrong, DDS, MS

Margherita Fontana, DDS, PhD

Marcelle M. Nascimento, DDS, MS, PhD

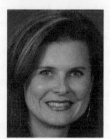

Andrea G. Ferreira Zandona, DDS, MSD, PhD

Editors

According to the World Health Organization, dental caries remains a major oral health problem in most industrialized countries, affecting 60% to 90% of schoolchildren and the vast majority of adults. Caries is the most prevalent oral disease causing major public health problems. The impact on individuals, families, and communities, as a result of pain and suffering, impairment of function, and reduced quality of life, is substantial. Moreover, the traditional surgical treatment for caries is extremely costly; it is

Dent Clin N Am 63 (2019) xiii–xv
https://doi.org/10.1016/j.cden.2019.07.003
0011-8532/19/© 2019 Published by Elsevier Inc.

dental.theclinics.com

the fourth most expensive disease to treat in most industrialized countries.[1] According to the Global Burden of Disease study in 2010, caries shares common risk factors with obesity and other noncommunicable diseases, such as cardiovascular diseases and diabetes.[2] Therefore, strategies to reduce the common risk factors for these diseases can improve the overall health of the population worldwide. Clearly, we cannot restore away the disease of caries, as managing the end point of this disease has not resulted in a decrease in caries prevalence. We must go beyond a surgical approach.

There is robust evidence that caries is a preventable disease; however, translating existing knowledge into practical and effective actions is a challenge. It is well known today that many behavioral and psychosocial factors can affect the lifestyle of an individual and family, and consequently, impact caries risk, treatment options, and clinical outcomes. Thus, management of caries in modern dentistry has evolved over decades from care of the patient by a single health care professional to care of the patient by a health care team. Interprofessional awareness and collaboration are essential to prevent and manage caries based on individual risk factors, and aid in decreasing disease disparities and enable access to care.

This issue of *Dental Clinics of North America* has the intent to provide an overall understanding of the impact that other health care providers have in the management of caries as well as the most current evidence associated with its cause and management. The current issue begins with the scientific principles of caries cause from the biofilm ecology perspective to dietary approaches on nutritional counseling. Subsequent articles offer updates on nonsurgical and surgical management of cavitated and noncavitated caries lesions and a framework to guide clinical decisions on how to implement strategies in a personalized manner.

Person-centered care and management focus on the elements of care, support, and treatment that matters most to the patient and their family, taking in consideration multiple factors.[3] Heath care providers, such as social workers, nurses, physicians, psychologists, and dieticians, have a critical role in the management of caries disease, and a continuous collaboration with appropriate referral is necessary. Thus, health and social services should be viewed as equal partners. "Building on the relationships with better communication in referrals, bidirectionally, reintegrates the mouth into the body and oral health into systemic health, with improvement in patient care and provider satisfaction" (Fisher-Owens).

Another aspect that challenges our profession and influences the management of caries is the financial system for oral health care. This is also discussed in this issue. Governments, payers, providers, and consumers are affected in different ways and should make meaningful progress in how caries management benefits are delivered and paid for in the future. Value models around the management of oral diseases should be a priority and an opportunity to reduce the long-term cost of treatments. The initial and long-term costs associated with the type of treatment used will have consequences in the overall health of the population and in many ways guide the providers' clinical decision making.

The ultimate goal of this issue is to provide an overall understanding of the influence of oral diseases in the overall health of our patients. Therefore, collaborating with other health care providers is essential.

Sandra Guzmán-Armstrong, DDS, MS
Operative Dentistry Department
University of Iowa
S-246 Dental Science Building
Iowa City, IA 52242-1001, USA

Margherita Fontana, DDS, PhD
Department of Cariology
Restorative Sciences & Endodontics
University of Michigan School of Dentistry
1011 North University, Room 2393
Ann Arbor, MI 48109-1078, USA

Marcelle M. Nascimento, DDS, MS, PhD
Department of Restorative Dental Sciences
University of Florida College of Dentistry
1395 Center Drive, Room D9-6
Gainesville, FL 32610-0415, USA

Andrea G. Ferreira Zandona, DDS, MSD, PhD
Department of Comprehensive Care
Tufts University School of Dental Medicine
1 Kneeland Street, Room 416
Boston, MA 02111, USA

E-mail addresses:
Sandra-guzman-armstrong@uiowa.edu (S. Guzmán-Armstrong)
mfontan@umich.edu (M. Fontana)
mnascimento@dental.ufl.edu (M.M. Nascimento)
Andrea.Zandona@tufts.edu (A.G. Ferreira Zandona)

REFERENCES

1. Righolt AJ, Jevdjevic M, Marcenes W, et al. Global-, regional-, and country-level economic impacts of dental diseases in 2015. J Dent Res 2018;97(5):501–7.
2. Marcenes W, Kassebaum NJ, Bernabe E, et al. Global burden of oral conditions in 1990-2010: a systematic analysis. J Dent Res 2013;92(7):592–7.
3. Walji MF, Karimbux NY, Spielman AI. Person-centered care: opportunities and challenges for academic dental institutions and programs. J Dent Educ 2017; 81(11):1265–72.

Approaches to Modulate Biofilm Ecology

Marcelle M. Nascimento, DDS, MS, PhD

KEYWORDS

• Dental caries • Oral health • pH • Plaque • Bacteria • Biofilm

KEY POINTS

• The pH and carbohydrate availability are key environmental factors affecting the physiology, ecology, and pathogenicity of oral biofilms colonizing teeth.
• Maintenance of oral health depends on the homeostasis of a consortium of commensal bacteria, such as that found in healthy-associated supragingival oral biofilms.
• Novel anticaries strategies include the modulation of the biofilm pH via arginine metabolism, nanotechnologies using acid-activated agents, oral probiotics and prebiotics, species-specific antimicrobial peptides targeting cariogenic pathogens, and other antibiofilm-specific approaches.

INTRODUCTION

After several decades of oral microbiology research, the scientific community has come to a simple conclusion - that a healthy mouth is a happy place to live if you are an oral commensal organism. In this context, the pH of supragingival oral biofilms is a key factor affecting the ecological "harmony" or homeostasis seen in oral heath. Oral commensals thrive at pH range between 6.0 and 7.0, which is the typical pH of resting biofilms colonizing healthy tooth surfaces. Advances in genome sequencing platforms, coupled with traditional microbiological studies, for analysis of the composition and function of the oral microbiome, have provided new insights in the etiology of oral diseses, and in particular, dental caries. Dental caries is closely related to a dysbiosis of the microbial consortia of supragingival biofilms driven by environmental changes, such as a sugar-frequent and acidic-pH environment. The concept of preventing the microbial dysbiosis related to caries through modulation of sugar intake and pH has fully emerged. Novel anti-caries strategies have been developed in recent years including modulation of the biofilm pH via arginine metabolism, nano

Disclosure Statement: Some of the author's research work cited in this article has been supported by the National Institute of Dental and Craniofacial Research and by Colgate-Palmolive.
Department of Restorative Dental Sciences, Division of Operative Dentistry, College of Dentistry, University of Florida, 1395 Center Drive, Room D9-6, PO Box 100415, Gainesville, FL 32610-0415, USA
E-mail address: mnascimento@dental.ufl.edu

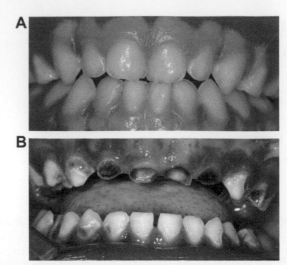

Fig. 1. (*A*) Child presenting a healthy oral cavity. (*B*) Child presenting early childhood dental caries (ECC). (*Courtesy of* Marcelle M. Nascimento, DDS, MS, PhD, Gainesville, FL.)

technologies using acidic-triggered anti-caries agents, oral probiotics and prebiotics, species-specific antimicrobial peptides targeting cariogenic pathogens, and synergistic combination of bacterial killing and extra polysaccharides (EPS) matrix digestion. Yet, deeper understanding of the mechanisms of action and toxicity of these new technologies using *in vivo* models and further efficacy validation in clinical studies are required. This chapter summarizes our current knowledge of the healthy oral microbiome and these exciting new technologies being developed to promote dental health.

The oral microbial ecosystem plays an essential role in human health. This is because the oral cavity is a major portal of microbial entry to the human body, and the altered oral microbiota has been intimately associated with oral and systemic diseases. The potential link between oral diseases (eg, dental caries and severe periodontitis) (**Figs. 1** and **2**) and systemic diseases (eg, cardiovascular disease, rheumatoid arthritis, and diabetes) has prompted great interest in the oral microbiome.[1,2] There is also an evolving trend for dental and medical research to share knowledge on the etiology and pathogenicity of human diseases.[3,4] Such interest follows insights provided from the Human Microbiome Project revealing that ecological balance in biofilms plays a significant role in health.[4]

Nowadays, ecologists and data scientists are beginning to collaborate with clinical scientists, and this teamwork is crucial to understand the potential of microbiome-informed and microbiome-based medicine and why not microbiome-based dentistry? Improvements in the throughput and accuracy of DNA sequencing of the genomes of microbial communities of human samples, accompanied by analysis of transcriptomes, proteomes, metabolomes, and immunomes, and by functional experiments, have vastly improved the ability to understand the structure and function of the microbiome associated with disease and health. Our understanding of the link between the oral and the human microbiome is rapidly expanding. In the era of applied meta-omics and personalized medicine, the oral microbiome is a valuable asset.[5] The oral microbiome encompasses the ecological community of commensal, symbiotic, and pathogenic microorganisms that share the mouth space.[6] This community forms a dynamic and complex microbial ecosystem that usually exists in homeostasis or symbiotic

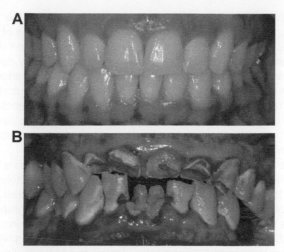

Fig. 2. (*A*) Adult presenting a healthy oral cavity. (*B*) Adult presenting both dental caries and periodontal diseases. (*Courtesy of* Marcelle M. Nascimento, DDS, MS, PhD, Gainesville, FL.)

state with the host, such as that found in healthy-associated supragingival oral biofilms.[7]

THE ECOLOGICAL COMPLEXITY OF THE HUMAN MOUTH

From the time of birth, the human mouth is a primary point of entry of microorganisms into the human body.[6] Microorganisms in the air food and those that are transferred through oral fluids (mainly saliva) from family members, caregivers, and others, can either just pass through the mouth or they can colonize the several oral niches. In fact, the complex ecosystem of the mouth supports the growth of diverse microbial communities comprising bacteria, viruses, mycoplasmas, archaea, fungi and protozoa that coinhabit and functionally interact in oral biofilms. The environmental factors that make the mouth such an attractive place for microorganisms include the: moisture and warmth (35°-37°C), presence of a variety of microbial niches, and abundance and continual influx of nutrients for microbial growth, such as salivary proteins, glycoproteins, and dietary components such as carbohydrates.[8,9] As a result, the human mouth is home to over 800 bacterial species organized into microbial communities that occupy multiple niches, including saliva, dental plaque, gingival crevice, and various soft tissue surfaces that compose the buccal mucosa and the tongue.[6]

The most abundant members of the oral microbiota are commensal organisms beneficial for oral health, but pathogens responsible for oral disease also exist. Commensal communities function to maintain the normal development of host tissues and defenses, by providing colonization resistance and down-regulation of damaging host inflammatory responses. However, the homeostasis or symbiotic relationship between the oral microbiome and the host is highly dynamic, as the composition and metabolic activities of microbial communities fluctuate according to the environmental changes in pH, nutrient availability, oxygen tension and redox environment, shedding effects of oral surfaces, and composition of salivary and crevicular fluids.[10]

The pH and carbohydrate availability are key environmental factors affecting the physiology, ecology, and pathogenicity of the oral biofilms colonizing the teeth.[11] Many beneficial oral bacteria can tolerate short periods of low pH, but their growth is inhibited by prolonged or frequent exposures to acidic conditions. In this context, the buffering activity of saliva plays a major role in maintaining the intraoral pH at around neutrality, which is optimal for the growth of most members of the oral microbiome.[12] Changes in environmental pH occur following consumption of dietary sugar. Specifically, organic acids produced by the fermentation of dietary carbohydrates by cariogenic bacteria elicit demineralization of tooth enamel. These periods of acid challenge to the tooth are followed by periods of alkalization, which neutralizes plaque pH and promotes remineralization of tooth enamel.[11] Whereas many factors contribute to the alkalization of oral biofilms (eg, buffers in saliva or diffusion of acids out of biofilms), alkali generation by oral bacteria plays a major role in pH homeostasis in oral biofilms and inhibits the initiation and progression of dental caries.[11,13,14]

Oral microorganisms gain substantial advantages by growing as a biofilm, and by functioning as a microbial community. Biofilms are inherently more tolerant to environmental stresses, host defenses, and antimicrobial agents, compared with growth as single microbial cells. The complex spatial organization or biogeography of supragingival oral biofilms was demonstrated by spectral imaging fluorescence in situ hybridization (CLASI-FISH) and metagenomic sequence analysis.[15] *Corynebacterium* was shown as the cornerstone of supragingival plaque architecture with long filaments that serve as anchor sites for many other microorganisms.[15] This study also revealed that individual taxa are localized at the micron scale, in ways suggestive of their functional niche in the biofilm consortium. For example, anaerobic taxa tend to be in the interior, whereas facultative or obligate aerobes tend to be at the periphery of the consortium. Consumers and producers of certain metabolites such as lactate (the main acid dissolving tooth tissues) tend to be near each other.

The architecture of oral biofilms allows for synergetic and antagonistic interactions among different microbial species, and these interactions are central to homeostasis. Genome sequencing techniques have identified some of these oral microorganisms, but several others - about one-third of oral bacteria - are yet to be isolated from oral samples and cultivated in the laboratory by using conventional microbiological methods. Bacterial cultivation of certain strains may be challenging, because of their specific requirements for nutrients, while others may be inhibited by substances in the culture media, or produced by other bacteria.[16] However, recent progress has been made on cultivating or cocultivating the so-called uncultivable bacteria, and greater knowledge about the ecological role of these "hard-to-grow bugs is being acquired.

THE CARIES MICROBIOME

The microbiome that naturally colonizes teeth in health is a biofilm community that can counterbalance acid production from dietary intake of carbohydrates to maintain an intact tooth surface (eg, by ammonia production from arginine or urea).[11] As proposed by Marsh,[17] excessive and frequent intake of carbohydrates exceeds the buffering capacity of the healthy microbiome and leads to dysbiosis of the biofilm with change of the bacterial composition (**Fig. 3**). Current knowledge points to a symbiotic relationship between the oral microbiome and the host in health, contrasting with a dysbiosis of the microbial consortia driven by a sugar-frequent and acidic -pH environment in dental caries.[18–20] In caries, continuous acid production from the metabolism of dietary carbohydrates favors the emergence of a highly acidogenic and aciduric microflora, enriched for *Streptococcus mutans*, other acid-tolerant streptococci, and *Lactobacillus* species. This selective process alters the pH homeostasis of supragingival biofilms and shifts the demineralization-remineralization equilibrium toward loss of tooth minerals.

Several studies support the observations that human supragingival dental plaque harbors a highly diverse bacterial community and that the microbiome of healthy tooth

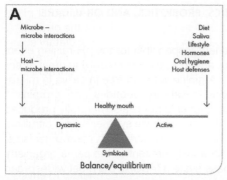
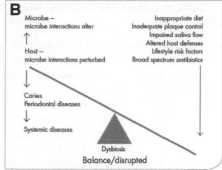

Fig. 3. A schematic representation of the dynamic relationship between the oral microbiome and the host environment in health and disease. (*A*) In health, a natural balance is maintained between host and environmental factors that results in a stable microbiota (ie, microbe-microbe interactions are in equilibrium), and a beneficial relationship with host tissues is established. This symbiotic relationship is susceptible to change. (*B*) A major change in the oral environment or lifestyle of the host can upset the delicate balance that exists among the many species that make up the oral microbiota. Previously minor components can become more competitive and predominate, which disrupts the previously symbiotic relationship with the host and increases the risk of disease. (Reprinted with permission from the California Dental Association, copyright October 2017.)[17]

surfaces differs substantially from that found when there is evidence of caries activity.[21–24] Changes in the microbial profile with the progressive stages of early childhood caries were observed when supragingival plaque of healthy tooth surfaces was compared with those of enamel and dentin carious lesions.[7] In particular, plaque communities from dentin carious lesions of caries-active children showed a distinctive bacterial profile compared with the other communities. Moreover, communities from healthy tooth surfaces of caries-active children (CA-PF) were shown to be more similar to those from enamel carious lesions (CAE-PE and CA-PE) than to those of healthy teeth from caries-free children (CF-PF); suggesting that CA-PF sites appear to be at greater risk of caries development than CF-PF sites. This finding is concordant with previous risk factor studies for childhood caries[25] and highlights the interconnectedness of plaque communities, in which these communities are part of a larger ecosystem where changes in the structure of 1 community may eventually affect others.

MODULATION OF BIOFILM pH

Carious lesions develop in tooth surfaces where there is an imbalance of the processes of acid and alkali production by supragingival biofilms. Because low pH is the main driving factor in the development of carious lesions, most efforts to identify an effective anticaries therapy have focused on targeting the acid-producing bacteria and their mechanisms of acid production. An expanding area of oral microbiology has been devoted to exploring microbial metabolic activities that help to neutralize biofilm pH, and thus inhibit the caries process. One way to restore biofilm homeostasis is to equilibrate the acidity and alkalinity processes in order to maintain a neutral biofilm pH. Physiologic factors that can counterbalance the acidification of biofilms include the clearance and buffering capacity of saliva and the metabolism of salivary substrates, such as urea and arginine, which generate alkali in the form of ammonia. In particular, ammonia production from arginine metabolism of oral bacteria inhibits tooth demineralization by neutralizing glycolytic acids and by favoring the growth of a desirable microflora that is compatible with dental health.[26]

ARGININE IN CARIES PREVENTION: PREBIOTICS, PROBIOTICS, AND ORAL CARE FORMULATIONS

L-arginine was identified as the main component responsible for the pH-raising effect of saliva by early in vitro studies,[27–29] and this amino acid is now receiving great attention because of its potential health benefits. Arginine is found free in saliva in micromolar concentrations, and is also abundant in salivary peptides and proteins.[30] Arginine enters the mouth through dietary components but is also naturally produced by the human body via protein turnover and de novo arginine synthesis from citrulline. Multiple pathways for arginine degradation have been described in microorganisms, and occasionally several of them are simultaneously present in the same organism. Among these pathways, the arginine deiminase system (ADS) is the most widespread anaerobic route for arginine degradation.[31]

In supragingival biofilms, arginine is metabolized mainly by ADS of certain oral bacteria to produce citrulline, ornithine, CO_2, ATP, and ammonia (**Fig. 4**). Ammonia production via ADS results in cytoplasmic and environment pH rises and serves as a mechanism used by oral bacteria for

- Protection against acid killing
- Bioenergetic advantages, including the increase of ΔpH and synthesis of ATP
- Maintaining a neutral environmental pH that favors the persistence of ADS-positive (ADS+) bacteria while being competitive against caries pathogens[11]

The potential for arginine metabolism to prevent caries has been supported by compelling evidence from in vitro studies[32–38] and clinical observations.[13,30,34] Salivary levels of free arginine are strongly correlated with caries resistance.[30] Plaque of caries-free individuals has higher pH values compared with plaque from caries-active individuals,[34,37,39] and this difference has been correlated with elevated ammonia levels in caries-free subjects.[34] The author's clinical studies revealed a positive correlation between caries activity and low arginolytic capacity of the supragingival microbial populations of adults and children.[13,14] In brief, the author and colleagues measured the ADS activity of plaque collected from caries-free tooth

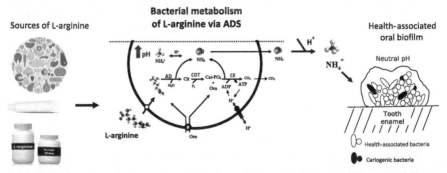

Fig. 4. Bacterial arginine metabolism via the ADS (arginine deiminase system), which is a 3-enzyme pathway (AD, arginine deiminase; COT, catabolic ornithine transcarbamylase; and CK, catabolic carbamate kinase). The major sources of arginine (L-arginine) for oral bacteria are: diet (fruits, vegetables, and animal sources), arginine as salivary peptides, de novo arginine synthesis from citrulline via protein turnover by the human body, use of oral care products (eg, toothpastes) and mints, and arginine supplements (eg, L-arginine capsules and protein shakes). Ammonia production via ADS results in increased pH values of the bacterial cytoplasmic and supragingival oral biofilms.

surfaces, enamel carious lesions, and dentin carious lesions of children who were either caries free or caries active.[14] Mixed-model analysis evaluated if age, type of dentition, children's caries status, and plaque caries status could be used as predictors of ADS activity. A recent cohort study revealed the arginolytic potential of supragingival plaque populations of children over time in the context of caries status.[40] As observed in previous cross-sectional studies, plaque bacteria from caries-free children and caries-free tooth surfaces had consistently higher ADS activity compared with those from caries-active children and carious tooth surfaces during the 18 months of the study ($P<.0001$).[40]

Numerous therapies have been proposed to target specific caries pathogens or indiscriminately eliminate oral biofilms (eg, xylitol, chlorhexidine,[41] immunization, and bacterial replacement therapy).[42] However, the effectiveness of these methods is yet to be recognized, and safety concerns have been raised with regards to their negative impact in the ecology of the oral microbiota. Novel therapies that seek to provide arginine as a substrate for ammonia production in oral biofilms may have high cost-effective potential for at-risk populations facing challenges accessing dental care. These promising approaches may include the use of arginine as prebiotic, selected ADS$^+$ strains as probiotic, and/or introduction of arginine in oral care formulations.

A technology designed to deliver arginine for ammonia production by plaque bacteria[43] has been incorporated into toothpastes, mints, and chews. Over the last 10 years, clinical trials have been conducted to evaluate the anticaries efficacy of products containing this original arginine technology or other optimized arginine formulations with or without fluoride.[44,45] A toothpaste containing 1.5% arginine, an insoluble calcium compound, and 1450 ppm of fluoride was also shown to reduce caries increments in low- and moderate-risk children, to arrest and reverse carious lesions in children and adults, and to have superior caries benefits compared with a regular toothpaste containing 1450 ppm of fluoride alone.[46] Thus, the mechanisms of action of arginine appear to complement those of fluoride by directly influencing biofilm pH while impacting the composition of oral biofilms. Even though the supplementation of arginine to oral biofilms can be effective against caries, the long-term impact of these novel arginine-based technologies on oral health and etiology of other oral diseases such as periodontal disease remains to be investigated.

ORAL PROBIOTICS FOR CARIES CONTROL

The use of orally administered probiotic species is gaining popularity as a strategy for maintaining oral health. Probiotics are defined as viable microorganisms that confer health benefits when administered in sufficient doses. There is a long history behind the use of probiotics for prevention and treatment of many medical conditions. Probiotics are an alternative to pharmaceutical management, notwithstanding the constant debates on their beneficial versus adverse effects. The increased popularity of using probiotic bacteria to improve gastrointestinal health has prompted interest in the value of this approach for oral applications. Consequently, much attention has been given lately to the role of probiotics in preventing caries, and the administration of different strains of *Lactobacilli* and/or *Bifidobacteria* has been tested to battle cariogenic bacteria.[47] The mechanisms of action of probiotics are thought to combine local and systemic effects including adhesion, coaggregation, growth inhibition, production of organic acids and bacteriocins, and immune modulation,[48] with the ultimate goal of displacing and perhaps replacing pathogens. These mechanisms may vary according to the specific bacterial strain or combinations of strains used, the delivery system, and the stage of the disease process in which the probiotic is administered.

Several studies have demonstrated successful in vivo and in vitro application of dairy product-derived oral probiotic species, predominantly lactobacilli, highlighting the potential of probiotics in oral health care. Select strains of lactobacilli inhibit growth and biofilm formation of caries-associated species *S. mutans* and *Candida albicans* in culture.[49] In vitro biofilm growth assays demonstrated that strains of *Lactobacillus, Lactococcus*, and *Streptococcus* can integrate into saliva-derived or defined-species biofilms and are maintained in the biofilms over several days.[48,50,51] However, an in vivo study reported that no probiotic lactobacilli were detected in dental plaque of individuals after 8-day treatment with fermented milk,[52] so the method by which such probiotic strains act on the biofilm in vivo needs further investigation.

Although the potential of using probiotics to manage caries appears to be high, the probiotic strains tested for oral health are, at the moment, microorganisms used mainly for gastrointestinal benefits, and they are likely not to adapt well to the unique environmental conditions and complex ecology of oral biofilms.[47] These probiotic strains do not seem to colonize the oral cavity permanently, which may be related to the number of receptors in the dental pellicle available for colonization of these nonoral strains compared with receptors for indigenous oral bacteria.[53] It has been proposed that naturally occurring oral strains with diminished cariogenic potential and desirable antagonistic properties on cariogenic bacteria may be proven successful as probiotic therapies for caries.[54] These oral species have the advantage of being adapted to growth in the mouth and the oral biofilm, and they may offer more sustainable and longer-term probiotic benefits than species from external sources like dairy products. In particular, several *Streptococcus* species, including *Streptococcus gordonii*, *Streptococcus sanguinis*, and *Streptococcus salivarius* are associated with oral health, and *S salivarius* K12 has been adapted as a probiotic for pharyngitis/tonsillitis, halitosis, and otitis media. In this context, *Streptococcus* A12 and other arginolytic clinical strains with constitutionally high ADS-expressing phenotypes and those capable of expressing ADS under conditions known to cause caries (eg, sugar availability and acidic environment) are being tested as probiotic strains for caries prevention.

PREBIOTICS FOR CARIES CONTROL

Prebiotics are defined as fermented food ingredients that can change the composition and/or activity of the resident microflora and confer benefits upon host well-being and health.[55] The concept of prebiotic has attracted and inspired research in many areas of nutrition and medical sciences. Several studies have shown that dietary consumption of certain food products can selectively modulate the indigenous composition of the gut microbiota.[56] However, sugars and dietary fiber, which are considered to be prebiotics for intestinal lactic acid bacteria, are not suited for the oral environment. Some potential oral prebiotics such as xylitol, xylose, and arabinose could suppress the growth of *S. mutans*, but they could also promote the growth of some lactobacilli strains. Given the lack of some suitable oral prebiotics, there several studies attempting to identify new prebiotics. As a natural dietary supplement, arginine has been extensively researched in medicine primarily to improve the symptoms of cardiovascular disease.[57] This is because arginine is a precursor of nitric oxide (NO), which plays important roles in vasodilatation, bacterial challenge and cytokine stimulation, regulation of mineralized tissue function, neurotransmission, and platelet aggregation.[58]

Recent in vitro studies have shown that providing L-arginine to supragingival biofilms disrupts the process of biofilm matrix assembly and the microbial interactions that are associated with the development of cariogenic biofilms,[59] and also confers biofilm pH homeostasis.[60] Interestingly, dietary questionnaires used in the author's clinical studies revealed that a group of caries-free participants presenting extremely high levels of plaque ADS activity reported high consumption of protein bars or protein shakes, which are major sources of arginine (Nascimento et al, unpublished data, 2019). Although arginine supplementation may have a positive impact in supragingival biofilms, NO generated from arginine metabolism may be involved in the pathogenesis of periodontitis.[61] Clearly, long-term randomized clinical trials are needed to determine whether dietary supplementation of arginine could be advantageous for oral health. Besides, it is critical to determine the correct supplementation level of dietary arginine before this amino acid can be used as a prebiotic approach for caries intervention.

ANTIBIOFILM TECHNOLOGIES USING pH AND OTHER ENVIRONMENTAL STIMULI

Triggering antibiofilm activity in response to pathogenic microenvironments could specifically target the development of cariogenic biofilms. Treating cariogenic biofilms is puzzling, as the organisms are often embedded in a protective, highly adherent, cohesive, and difficult to remove EPS matrix. Conventional antimicrobial modalities are limited in addressing the biochemical properties of the biofilm matrix, whereas upcoming therapeutic strategies are being developed to specifically target the microenvironments of the matrix and the embedded bacteria with minimal cytotoxicity to surrounding tissues. Nanotechnologies that can penetrate biofilms and damage the matrix may enhance antibacterial efficacy and minimize initiation of drug or antibacterial resistance.

Functional polymeric nanostructures (PNs) were developed for enhanced drug delivery when triggered by acidic pH values.[62] These nanostructures are formed from diblock copolymers and 2-propylacrylic acid that self-assemble into cationic nanoparticles, and they have adsorption affinities to salivary pellicle and EPS-coated apatitic surfaces because of strong electrostatic interaction.[62] In addition, the nanoparticles endure core destabilization and drug release in response to changes in pH, triggered by biofilm acidification.

Another promising approach employs pH-responsive catalytic inorganic nanoparticles (CAT-NPs) with antibiofilm and anticaries properties.[63] Nanoparticles containing biocompatible iron-oxide (Fe_3O_4) with peroxidase-like activity were developed to catalyze H_2O_2 in a pH-dependent manner (eg, greater catalytic activity at low pH and no activity at neutral pH).[64] In situ studies showed that under acidic pH, the catalytic nanoparticles can generate free radicals from H_2O_2 that concurrently damage the EPS matrix and kill the biofilm bacteria within 5 minutes.[64] CAT-NPs were also shown to decrease demineralization of apatite disks in vitro. CAT-NPs in combination with H_2O_2 were tested in vivo as 1-minute topical daily treatments, and the results were shown to decrease caries development without harmful effects to soft tissues.[64] Further toxicity studies are needed to investigate the long-term effects of topical applications, but the combination of CAT-NPs and H_2O_2 has clinical potential.

APPROACHES TO DISRUPT BIOFILMS

Other recent approaches have emerged to disrupt the biofilm microbial composition and the microenvironment.[65] An S. mutans-specific targeting approach was developed using synthetic antimicrobial peptide (AMP) consisting of dual-functionally independent moieties (named C16G2), a broad-spectrum, novispirin-derived AMP killing region (G2) attached to an S. mutans-specific peptide pheromone that provides targeting specificity (C16).[65] Selective killing of S. mutans was achieved after increased rate of G2 accumulation on the bacterial surface. In this study, the population of S. mutans was reduced from multispecies biofilm communities, while the abundance of commensal streptococci, including Streptococcus mitis, Streptococcus oralis, and S sanguinis were increased.[65] An AMP containing an S. mutans-targeting domain to the ComC signaling peptide fused with a killing domain composed of broad-spectrum AMP pleurocidin was also demonstrated to enhance specificity against S. mutans while maintaining S sanguinis or S gordonii cells in vitro.[66] This is another example of a targeted killing approach, which may remove specific pathogens from cariogenic biofilms to promote a healthy-like microbiome. However, and as mentioned for all approaches cited previously, in vivo studies are necessary to better understand the anticaries mechanisms and efficacy as well as to address safety concerns.

Biopharmaceuticals made via plant-chloroplast technology are also being considered as a biofilm-disrupting approach for caries control. The US Food and Drug Administration (FDA) approval of plant-produced protein drugs supports the clinical advancement of this type pf technology. For example, an approach using plant-made antimicrobial peptide (PMAMP)-Protegrin (PG1) was also developed for topical use to control biofilms.[67,68] PMAMP-PG1 was shown to rapidly killed S. mutans and impaired biofilm formation following a single topical application of the tooth-mimetic apatite surface. The combined use of PG1 with 2 EPS-degrading enzymes, dextranase and mutanase, was capable of digesting biofilm matrix and facilitating peptide access into the biofilm structure in addition to killing bacterial clusters.[68,69]

WHERE ARE WE HEADING?

Future research precisely identifying the key oral microbiota in health and disease will contribute to the advancement of more effective tools for modulation of oral biofilms. Even though the healthy oral microbiome appears to be more stable than those of other body niches like the gut, there is evidence for a substantial degree of within-individual variability in the oral microbiome.[70,71] Genetic diversity and complexities in the adaptive strategies of oral bacteria to fluctuating biofilm conditions diminish the utility of taxa-level correlation of the microbiome with health especially, but also with caries and periodontal disease. The relevant questions may be answered by elucidating what the microbes are doing, rather than focusing primarily on what is performing those actions.[20] Also deserving more attention are the microbial interactions with the host (eg, adhesion mechanisms between microbes and salivary proteins)[72] and the recognition patterns with the oral immune system.[73] Future directions should focus on achieving maximal efficacy and targeting specificity with minimal toxicity and long-term therapeutic effects. These, along with enhanced drug delivery/activation within pathogenic microenvironments, may enlighten the way for an effective therapeutic strategy with high precision against cariogenic biofilms.

SUMMARY

Studies of the oral microbiome may hold the answers for understanding human diseases even beyond the oral cavity. Several emerging strategies for modulation of supragingival oral biofilms have been explored and are being successfully developed and tested in vitro. Still, clinical studies are needed to investigate the efficacy and safety of these approaches for caries prevention and control. Future microbiome and metagenome analyses will certainly contribute to the development of more effective therapeutic and diagnostic techniques and ultimately to personalized medicine and personalized dentistry.

REFERENCES

1. Cahill TJ, Harrison JL, Jewell P, et al. Antibiotic prophylaxis for infective endocarditis: a systematic review and meta-analysis. Heart 2017;103(12):937–44.
2. Kriebel K, Hieke C, Muller-Hilke B, et al. Oral biofilms from symbiotic to pathogenic interactions and associated disease -connection of periodontitis and rheumatic arthritis by peptidylarginine deiminase. Front Microbiol 2018;9:53.
3. Proctor LM. The National Institutes of Health human microbiome project. Semin Fetal Neonatal Med 2016;21(6):368–72.
4. Turnbaugh PJ, Ley RE, Hamady M, et al. The human microbiome project. Nature 2007;449(7164):804–10.
5. Gomez A, Nelson KE. The oral microbiome of children: development, disease, and implications beyond oral health. Microb Ecol 2017;73(2):492–503.
6. Dewhirst FE, Chen T, Izard J, et al. The human oral microbiome. J Bacteriol 2010; 192(19):5002–17.
7. Richards VP, Alvarez AJ, Luce AR, et al. Microbiomes of site-specific dental plaques from children with different caries status. Infect Immun 2017;85(8) [pii: e00106-17].
8. Jakubovics NS. Saliva as the sole nutritional source in the development of multispecies communities in dental plaque. Microbiol Spectr 2015;3(3):1–11.
9. Wei GX, van der Hoeven JS, Smalley JW, et al. Proteolysis and utilization of albumin by enrichment cultures of subgingival microbiota. Oral Microbiol Immunol 1999;14(6):348–51.
10. Burne RA, Zeng L, Ahn SJ, et al. Progress dissecting the oral microbiome in caries and health. Adv Dent Res 2012;24(2):77–80.
11. Burne RA, Marquis RE. Alkali production by oral bacteria and protection against dental caries. FEMS Microbiol Lett 2000;193(1):1–6.
12. Marsh PD, Takahashi N, Nyvad B. Biofilms in caries development. In: Fejerskov O, Nyvad B, Kidd E, editors. Dental caries: the disease and its clinical management. 3rd edition. Wiley-Blackwell; 2015. p. 107–31.
13. Nascimento MM, Gordan VV, Garvan CW, et al. Correlations of oral bacterial arginine and urea catabolism with caries experience. Oral Microbiol Immunol 2009; 24(2):89–95.
14. Nascimento MM, Liu Y, Kalra R, et al. Oral arginine metabolism may decrease the risk for dental caries in children. J Dent Res 2013;92(7):604–8.
15. Mark Welch JL, Rossetti BJ, Rieken CW, et al. Biogeography of a human oral microbiome at the micron scale. Proc Natl Acad Sci U S A 2016;113(6):E791–800.
16. Wade W, Thompson H, Rybalka A. Uncultured members of the oral microbiome. J Calif Dent Assoc 2016;44(7):447–56.
17. Marsh PD. Ecological events in oral health and disease: new opportunities for prevention and disease control? J Calif Dent Assoc 2017;45(10):525–37.
18. Marsh PD. Dental plaque as a biofilm and a microbial community - implications for health and disease. BMC Oral Health 2006;6(Suppl 1):S14.
19. Nascimento MM, Zaura E, Mira A, et al. Second era of OMICS in caries research: moving past the phase of disillusionment. J Dent Res 2017;96(7):733–40, 22034517701902.
20. Takahashi N. Oral microbiome metabolism: from "who are they?" to "what are they doing?". J Dent Res 2015;94(12):1628–37.
21. Aas JA, Griffen AL, Dardis SR, et al. Bacteria of dental caries in primary and permanent teeth in children and young adults. J Clin Microbiol 2008;46(4):1407–17.

22. Belda-Ferre P, Alcaraz LD, Cabrera-Rubio R, et al. The oral metagenome in health and disease. ISME J 2012;6(1):46–56.

23. Gross EL, Beall CJ, Kutsch SR, et al. Beyond *Streptococcus mutans*: dental caries onset linked to multiple species by 16S rRNA community analysis. PLoS One 2012;7(10):e47722.

24. Gross EL, Leys EJ, Gasparovich SR, et al. Bacterial 16S sequence analysis of severe caries in young permanent teeth. J Clin Microbiol 2010;48(11):4121–8.

25. Lee HJ, Kim JB, Jin BH, et al. Risk factors for dental caries in childhood: a five-year survival analysis. Community Dent Oral Epidemiol 2015;43(2):163–71.

26. Nascimento MM, Burne RA. Caries prevention by arginine metabolism in oral biofilms: translating science into clinical success. Curr Oral Health Rep 2014;1(1): 79–85.

27. Kanapka JA, Kleinberg I. Catabolism of arginine by the mixed bacteria in human salivary sediment under conditions of low and high glucose concentration. Arch Oral Biol 1983;28(11):1007–15.

28. Kleinberg I, Kanapka JA, Chatterjee R, et al. Metabolism of nitrogen by the oral mixed bacteria. London: Information Retrieval; 1979.

29. Wijeyeweera RL, Kleinberg I. Acid-base pH curves in vitro with mixtures of pure cultures of human oral microorganisms. Arch Oral Biol 1989;34(1):55–64.

30. Van Wuyckhuyse BC, Perinpanayagam HE, Bevacqua D, et al. Association of free arginine and lysine concentrations in human parotid saliva with caries experience. J Dent Res 1995;74(2):686–90.

31. Zuniga M, Perez G, Gonzalez-Candelas F. Evolution of arginine deiminase (ADI) pathway genes. Mol Phylogenet Evol 2002;25(3):429–44.

32. Imfeld T, Birkhed D, Lingstrom P. Effect of urea in sugar-free chewing gums on pH recovery in human dental plaque evaluated with three different methods. Caries Res 1995;29(3):172–80.

33. Kleinberg I. Prevention and dental caries. J Prev Dent 1978;5(3):9–17.

34. Margolis HC, Duckworth JH, Moreno EC. Composition of pooled resting plaque fluid from caries-free and caries-susceptible individuals. J Dent Res 1988; 67(12):1468–75.

35. Sissons CH, Cutress TW. pH changes during simultaneous metabolism of urea and carbohydrate by human salivary bacteria in vitro. Arch Oral Biol 1988; 33(8):579–87.

36. Kleinberg I. A mixed-bacteria ecological approach to understanding the role of the oral bacteria in dental caries causation: an alternative to *Streptococcus mutans* and the specific-plaque hypothesis. Crit Rev Oral Biol Med 2002;13(2): 108–25.

37. Stephan RM. Intra-oral hydrogen-ion concentration associated with dental caries activity. J Dent Res 1944;23:257–66.

38. Turtola LO, Luoma H. Plaque pH in caries-active and inactive subjects modified by sucrose and fluoride, with and without bicarbonate-phosphate. Scand J Dent Res 1972;80(4):334–43.

39. Rosen S, Weisenstein PR. The effect of sugar solutions on pH of dental plaques from caries-susceptible and caries-free individuals. J Dent Res 1965;44(5): 845–9.

40. Nascimento MM, Alvarez AJ, Huang X, et al. Arginine metabolism in supragingival oral biofilms as a potential predictor of caries risk. JDR Clin Trans Res 2019; 4(3):262–70, 2380084419834234.

41. James P, Parnell C, Whelton H. The caries-preventive effect of chlorhexidine varnish in children and adolescents: a systematic review. Caries Res 2010;44(4): 333–40.
42. Hillman JD. Genetically modified *Streptococcus mutans* for the prevention of dental caries. Antonie Van Leeuwenhoek 2002;82(1–4):361–6.
43. Kleinberg I. A new saliva-based anti-caries composition. Dent Today 1999;18: 98–103.
44. Acevedo AM, Machado C, Rivera LE, et al. The inhibitory effect of an arginine bicarbonate/calcium carbonate CaviStat-containing dentifrice on the development of dental caries in Venezuelan school children. J Clin Dent 2005;16(3):63–70.
45. Acevedo AM, Montero M, Rojas-Sanchez F, et al. Clinical evaluation of the ability of CaviStat in a mint confection to inhibit the development of dental caries in children. J Clin Dent 2008;19(1):1–8.
46. Kraivaphan P, Amornchat C, Triratana T, et al. Two-year caries clinical study of the efficacy of novel dentifrices containing 1.5% arginine, an insoluble calcium compound and 1,450 ppm fluoride. Caries Res 2013;47(6):582–90.
47. Cagetti MG, Mastroberardino S, Milia E, et al. The use of probiotic strains in caries prevention: a systematic review. Nutrients 2013;5(7):2530–50.
48. Devine DA, Marsh PD. Prospects for the development of probiotics and prebiotics for oral applications. J Oral Microbiol 2009;1:1–11.
49. Hasslof P, West CE, Videhult FK, et al. Early intervention with probiotic *Lactobacillus paracasei* F19 has no long-term effect on caries experience. Caries Res 2013;47(6):559–65.
50. Twetman S, Keller MK. Probiotics for caries prevention and control. Adv Dent Res 2012;24(2):98–102.
51. Jindal G, Pandey RK, Agarwal J, et al. A comparative evaluation of probiotics on salivary mutans streptococci counts in Indian children. Eur Arch Paediatr Dent 2011;12(4):211–5.
52. Ravn I, Dige I, Meyer RL, et al. Colonization of the oral cavity by probiotic bacteria. Caries Res 2012;46(2):107–12.
53. Comelli EM, Guggenheim B, Stingele F, et al. Selection of dairy bacterial strains as probiotics for oral health. Eur J Oral Sci 2002;110(3):218–24.
54. Hillman JD, McDonell E, Cramm T, et al. A spontaneous lactate dehydrogenase deficient mutant of *Streptococcus rattus* for use as a probiotic in the prevention of dental caries. J Appl Microbiol 2009;107(5):1551–8.
55. Roberfroid M. Prebiotics: the concept revisited. J Nutr 2007;137(3 Suppl 2): 830S–7S.
56. Roberfroid M, Gibson GR, Hoyles L, et al. Prebiotic effects: metabolic and health benefits. Br J Nutr 2010;104(Suppl 2):S1–63.
57. Lorin J, Zeller M, Guilland JC, et al. Arginine and nitric oxide synthase: regulatory mechanisms and cardiovascular aspects. Mol Nutr Food Res 2014;58(1):101–16.
58. Morris SM Jr. Arginine metabolism revisited. J Nutr 2016;146(12):2579S–86S.
59. He J, Hwang G, Liu Y, et al. L-arginine modifies the exopolysaccharides matrix and thwarts *Streptococcus mutans* outgrowth within mixed-species oral biofilms. J Bacteriol 2016;198(19):2651–61.
60. Agnello M, Cen L, Tran NC, et al. Arginine improves pH homeostasis via metabolism and microbiome modulation. J Dent Res 2017;96(8):924–30.
61. Parwani SR, Parwani RN. Nitric oxide and inflammatory periodontal disease. Gen Dent 2015;63(2):34–40.

62. Horev B, Klein MI, Hwang G, et al. pH-activated nanoparticles for controlled topical delivery of farnesol to disrupt oral biofilm virulence. ACS Nano 2015; 9(3):2390–404.
63. Liu Y, Ren Z, Hwang G, et al. Therapeutic strategies targeting cariogenic biofilm microenvironment. Adv Dent Res 2018;29(1):86–92.
64. Gao L, Liu Y, Kim D, et al. Nanocatalysts promote *Streptococcus mutans* biofilm matrix degradation and enhance bacterial killing to suppress dental caries in vivo. Biomaterials 2016;101:272–84.
65. Guo L, McLean JS, Yang Y, et al. Precision-guided antimicrobial peptide as a targeted modulator of human microbial ecology. Proc Natl Acad Sci U S A 2015; 112(24):7569–74.
66. Mai J, Tian XL, Gallant JW, et al. A novel target-specific, salt-resistant antimicrobial peptide against the cariogenic pathogen *Streptococcus mutans*. Antimicrob Agents Chemother 2011;*55*(11):*5205–13.*
67. Liu L, Hao T, Xie Z, et al. Genome mining unveils widespread natural product biosynthetic capacity in human oral microbe *Streptococcus mutans*. Sci Rep 2016;6:37479.
68. Liu Y, Kamesh AC, Xiao Y, et al. Topical delivery of low-cost protein drug candidates made in chloroplasts for biofilm disruption and uptake by oral epithelial cells. Biomaterials 2016;105:156–66.
69. Kwon KC, Daniell H. Low-cost oral delivery of protein drugs bioencapsulated in plant cells. Plant Biotechnol J 2015;13(8):1017–22.
70. Caporaso JG, Lauber CL, Costello EK, et al. Moving pictures of the human microbiome. Genome Biol 2011;12(5):R50.
71. Turnbaugh PJ, Hamady M, Yatsunenko T, et al. A core gut microbiome in obese and lean twins. Nature 2009;457(7228):480–4.
72. Nobbs AH, Jenkinson HF, Jakubovics NS. Stick to your gums: mechanisms of oral microbial adherence. J Dent Res 2011;90(11):1271–8.
73. Simon-Soro A, Mira A. Solving the etiology of dental caries. Trends Microbiol 2015;23(2):76–82.

Dietary Implications for Dental Caries

A Practical Approach on Dietary Counseling

Teresa A. Marshall, PhD, RDN/LDN

KEYWORDS

- Diet • Caries • Sugar-sweetened beverages • Sugars • Diet assessment
- Diet counseling

KEY POINTS

- Dental caries is a diet-related disease; a healthy diet and eating behaviors form the foundation of caries prevention.
- Frequent and/or prolonged intakes of foods or beverages containing added sugars increase the risk of dental caries.
- Screening and assessing diet-related caries risk factors is part of the caries management process.
- Dietary counseling to reduce caries risk includes patient education as well as anticipatory guidance to improve patient health.

INTRODUCTION

Acid produced during bacterial fermentation of dietary carbohydrates dissolves enamel and/or dentin, leading to dental caries. Thus, caries is a diet-related disease. Although attention typically focuses on fermentable carbohydrates, specifically sugars, fermentable carbohydrates are not consumed in isolation. Carbohydrates are nutrients within foods and beverages. Individual foods and beverages contain a myriad of differing nutrients in varying concentrations, and ultimately food and beverage choices and eating behaviors are associated with the caries process. Consideration of food and beverage choices and eating behaviors is necessary for effective caries prevention. This article defines a healthy diet and eating behaviors as a foundation for caries prevention; identifies food and beverage choices and eating behaviors associated with caries; identifies diet-related screening and assessment tools for caries risk; and provides counseling strategies for patients at risk for dental caries.

Disclosure Statement: The author has nothing to disclose.
Department of Preventive and Community Dentistry, University of Iowa College of Dentistry, 335 Dental Science North, Iowa City, IA 52242-1010, USA
E-mail address: teresa-marshall@uiowa.edu

DIET

The term "diet" is simply defined as the foods and beverages one typically consumes. Foods and beverages deliver nutrients, which are defined as substances necessary for growth, maintenance, and/or repair of body tissues. Nutrients providing energy include proteins, fats, and carbohydrates. The terms "nutrient dense" and "energy dense" are used to describe the relative concentrations of nutrients and energy within individual foods and beverages. In addition to caries, the choice of foods and beverages consumed, balanced by their nutrient and energy densities, influences systemic health and chronic disease.

Dietary guidelines, including the United States Dietary Guidelines (USDG), offer recommendations for health promotion and disease prevention.[1] The overall objectives of dietary guidelines are to identify nutrients necessary for growth, maintenance, and repair; to recommend the types and amounts of foods to provide necessary nutrients; and to identify non-nutrient compounds or foods to limit for prevention of chronic disease. Recommended nutrient intakes are defined by age and gender in the Dietary Reference Intakes (DRIs).[2] Ideally, individuals choose nutrient-dense foods to meet their individual nutrient requirements within their energy requirements. Nutrients within foods are more bioavailable than nutrients from supplements; notable exceptions include vitamins B_{12} and folate.[3]

A healthy diet will limit exposure to excessive nutrient intakes, non-nutrient compounds associated with chronic disease (ie, added sugars, cholesterol), and environmental contaminates that might include lead, bacteria (ie, *Salmonella*), natural toxicants (ie, solanin), or pesticide exposures. The Tolerable Upper Intake Level within the DRIs identifies the maximum amount of a nutrient that is considered safe for most healthy individuals and beyond which there is an increased risk of adverse health effects by age and gender.[2] The USDG and the World Health Organization (WHO), respectively, recommend that intake of both added and free sugars be limited to less than 10% of total energy intake (ie, 12 teaspoons/2000 kcal) for oral and systemic health, with the WHO suggesting that 5% (ie, 6 teaspoons/2000 kcal) might be more appropriate for caries prevention.[1,4] Added sugars are defined as sugars used as ingredients and added during food processing, home preparation, or at the time of consumption, whereas free sugars are defined as sugars added to foods by the manufacturer, cook, or consumer or naturally present in honey, syrups, fruit juices, and fruit concentrates.[5,6] Inclusion of added sugar content on food labels is designed to help consumers make healthier food choices. In 2016, the United States Food and Drug Administration announced that grams of added sugars would be included on food labels beginning in 2018; implementation has been delayed until January 2020 for manufacturers with $10 million in food sales.[7]

Dietary guidelines throughout the world support consumption of minimally processed foods, particularly those readily available and accessible to the consumer. Minimally processed foods may have been cleaned, cooked, or preserved, and their origin is easily recognized.[8] By contrast, ultraprocessed foods are made from transformed food ingredients with little semblance to their original foodstuff (ie, chocolate, chips, hotdogs).[8] As the food commodity moves along the processing continuum, nutrient density decreases while energy density increases. The USDG generally recommends consumption of minimally processed foods, recognizing that limited quantities of ultraprocessed foods may be consumed within a healthy diet. ChooseMyPlate is an online program that translates the USDG to consumer food recommendations, and presents food group plans by age and gender for healthy Americans.[9] **Table 1** provides examples of ChooseMyPlate plans for males and females aged 4 to 8, 14 to 18, and 31 to 50 years, and is available at https://www.choosemyplate.gov/MyPlate.

The USDG and ChooseMyPlate are evidence based, and the science defining a healthy diet is clear. In reality, one's food choices are heavily influenced by multiple factors and not necessarily consistent with a healthy diet. The Social-Ecological Model is a visual framework that identifies individual, setting, sector, and social or cultural factors that influence food and activity decisions.[1] From a pragmatic perspective, transportation, finances, and living conditions heavily influence access to and availability of healthy food. Compliance with the USDG depends on a supportive environment; individuals of lower socioeconomic status often lack transportation to access the resources to purchase, and household facilities to safely store and prepare minimally processed foods.

EATING BEHAVIORS

Eating behaviors or habits refer to the when, where, and how foods and beverages are consumed. Although eating behaviors are known to influence food choices and systemic health, the science associating eating behaviors with caries risk is more advanced. In essence, eating behaviors that increase either the frequency or length of carbohydrate consumption will consequently increase the exposure time (ie, the opportunity for oral bacteria to ferment the carbohydrate), and thus increase the risk of caries.

The ideal eating behaviors match food and beverage intake to appropriate hunger cues. A mismatch between eating and hunger leading to prolonged or excessive hunger increases the risk of binge eating upon food or beverage presentation, and eating without hunger increases the likelihood of snacking on highly palatable, ultraprocessed foods or beverages at the expense of minimally processed foods. Thus, healthy eating behaviors emphasize structured eating and include 3 meals and 2 to 3 snacks per day. All energy-containing foods and beverages should be consumed within these structured eating events.

Young children have proportionately higher energy requirements than adults and smaller stomach capacities. For young children to consume adequate energy and nutrients, more frequent eating events are required. In addition, regular access to meals and snacks at appropriate intervals during early childhood is associated with food

Table 1
ChooseMyPlate daily food group plans for males and females aged 4–8, 14–18, and 31–50 years old

Food Group	Age 4–8 y Males and Females	Age 14–18 y Males	Age 14–18 y Females	Age 31–50 y Males	Age 31–50 y Females
Fruits (cups)	1–1.5	2.0	1.5	2.0	1.5
Vegetables (cups)	1.5	3.0	2.5	3.0	2.5
Grains (ounces)[a]	5	8.0	6.0	7.0	6.0
Protein foods (ounces)	4	6.5	5.0	6.0	5.0
Dairy (cups)	2.5	3.0	3.0	3.0	3.0
Oils (teaspoons)	4	6.0	5.0	6.0	5.0

[a] Half of daily grain recommendation should be whole grain.

Data from the United States Department of Agriculture. ChooseMyPlate.gov. Available at: https://www.choosemyplate.gov/MyPlate. Accessed 10/3/18.

security and a healthy relationship with food.[10] In adults, systemic conditions that alter stomach capacity and/or satiety responses might also affect the frequency of eating events.

Dietary recommendations for caries prevention should be consistent with age-appropriate eating behaviors and should consider systemic modifiers. From birth through 6 months of age, human milk and/or infant formula should be provided on demand in response to infant hunger cues. At approximately 6 months of age, texture-appropriate solid foods and meal structure should be introduced. By 1 year of age, all energy-containing foods and beverages should be provided at 3 meals and 2 to 3 snacks. The ubiquitous availability of foods and beverages within contemporary environments is associated with a decrease in structured eating events. Grazing or prolonged snacking on foods and/or beverages is commonplace. Unfortunately, the prolonged consumption of foods and/or beverages containing added sugars increases the opportunity for their fermentation within the oral cavity and subsequent caries risk.

Cultural customs that encourage or support the use of foods and/or beverages to address emotional needs can result in prolonged fermentable carbohydrate exposures that increase the risk of caries. Provision of minimally processed foods and/or beverages at gatherings to celebrate religious, cultural, or life events is a foundation of and central to many westernized celebrations. Indeed, children and adolescents raised in families sharing 3 or more meals per week are less likely to be overweight and more likely to eat healthy foods than peers sharing less than 3 meals.[11] However, the use of ultraprocessed foods and/or beverages to reward behaviors, heal wounds, or soften losses can lead to unhealthy relationships with foods,[12] which can lead to emotional eating—that is, using food to address emotional needs instead of using more appropriate means of dealing with emotions. Emotional eating is associated with unhealthy food choices and prolonged eating, both of which can increase the risk of dental caries.

DIET-RELATED CARIES RISK

The caries risk attributable to dietary factors is influenced by both food choices and eating behaviors. A continuum of caries risk is associated with each; for example, the summary of one's food choices might range from minimally processed with few added sugars to ultraprocessed with excessive added sugars. Likewise, eating behaviors might range from few to numerous episodes as well as from short to prolonged events. These 3 factors—added sugar intake, eating frequency, and length of eating event—interact to determine an individual's diet-associated caries risk. An individual whose added sugar intake is less than 5% of their total energy is likely to carry a low caries risk regardless of frequency or duration of eating events. Similarly, an individual with 1 or 2 short eating events per day is likely to be at low caries risk regardless of added sugar intake. Identification of risk becomes more complicated for individuals with moderate sugar intakes and frequent and/or prolonged eating events. Individuals with high added sugar intakes (>15% total energy) and frequent and/or prolonged eating events are at high dietary risk of caries, although good oral hygiene behaviors would likely reduce caries risk.

SCREENING AND ASSESSMENT OF DIET-RELATED CARIES RISK

All patients should be screened for diet-related caries risk, and those with positive screen responses or caries activity should receive an in-depth diet-related caries risk assessment.[13] A diet-related caries risk screen is designed to identify individuals whose food choices and/or eating behaviors place them at increased caries risk (**Table 2**). The goal of screening is to identify the risk, and intervene before the caries process becomes apparent. A diet-related caries risk assessment is designed to identify specific high-risk food choices and/or eating behaviors as well as overall dietary practices (**Table 3**). The goal of assessment is to identify alternative food choices and/or eating behaviors to decrease caries risk in the context of a nutritionally adequate diet. Knowledge of overall dietary practices is necessary to develop acceptable dietary recommendations with appropriate anticipatory guidance to reduce caries risk.

The desired outcome of diet-related caries risk recommendations is to decrease caries risk while maintaining adequate nutrient and energy intakes for normal growth, development, and activity.

COUNSELING

Preventing caries begins with education through communicating the risks associated with ultraprocessed foods containing added sugars and frequent and/or prolonged eating events. Food choices and eating behaviors associated with increased caries risk are also associated with obesity and obesity-related chronic diseases.[14] Thus, communicating the systemic health concerns of food choices to patients in addition

Table 2
Diet-related caries risk screen

Number	Question	Rationale	Potential Action
1	Do you drink sugar-sweetened beverages (SSBs) daily?	Concentrated source of added sugars; dietary risk factor for caries	
	a. If yes, how much do you drink each day?		If intake is greater than age-appropriate recommendations (see **Table 5**), then complete diet-related caries risk assessment Reduce intake to less than age-appropriate recommendations (see **Table 5**); drink at one event per day in <30 min If SSBs are caffeinated, then provide guidance to replace caffeine and/or gradually reduce caffeine intake
2	How many meals and/or snacks do you eat each day?	Increased frequency of eating increases caries risk	If more than 6 eating events after age 1–2 y of age, then complete diet-related caries risk assessment
3	Would you describe your eating patterns as structured (ie, meals and snacks at about the same times each day) or unstructured (ie, eating off and on throughout the day)?	Unstructured eating increases caries risk and is associated with lower diet quality	If unstructured, then complete diet-related caries risk assessment

Table 3
Diet-related caries risk assessment

Number	Question	Rationale	Potential Action
1	Are you following a special diet?	Background for diet-related recommendations	Diet-related caries risk recommendations should be consistent with systemic dietary recommendations
		Identify caries risk associated with special diet	Address food choices and eating behaviors associated with caries risk
2	What changes have you made to your diet during the past 6 months to a year?	Dietary changes might have implications for caries risk	Reinforce dietary changes that decrease caries risk and/or improve overall diet quality
			Address dietary changes that increase caries risk and/or decrease overall diet quality
3	24 h/usual recall: I'd like to know what you typically eat or drink each day. Starting after you woke up yesterday (or usually wake up), what did you have to eat or drink? *Prompt to continue throughout the day*	Identify food choices and eating patterns that increase caries risk	Identify current food preferences and behaviors, and note areas where patient might be receptive to change
		Knowledge of current food preferences and behaviors is the foundation for dietary recommendations	
	From patient description:		
	a. If meal patterns are not obvious from 24 h/usual recall, then ask about structure, frequency, and length of eating events	Meal patterns—structured to decrease caries risk	Guidance to increase structure (3 meals, 2–3 snacks), decrease frequency and length of eating events
	b. If SSBs, candies, pastries, or salty snacks are not mentioned during 24 h recall, then ask about each item	Ultraprocessed foods—SSBs, candies, pastries, or salty snacks increase caries risk	Limit SSB intake to age-appropriate guidelines (see **Table 5**) Limit candies, pastries, and salty snacks to structured eating events and occasional consumption
	c. If each food group is not mentioned during 24 h recall, then ask about the missing food groups	Food group intakes—minimally processed foods from all groups provide adequate nutrient intakes and displace ultraprocessed foods	First, encourage consumption of all food groups Second, encourage ChooseMyPlate quantities of all food groups
4	Do you have transportation (car or bus) to get to a store to purchase the foods you'd like to eat?	Identify access barriers to obtaining food	Refer to local agencies for assistance in obtaining food

(continued on next page)

Table 3
(continued)

Number	Question	Rationale	Potential Action
5	Do you have money and/or SNAP (Supplemental Nutritional Assistance Program) or other food benefits to purchase the foods you'd like to eat?	Identify access barriers to obtaining food	Refer to local agencies for assistance in obtaining food
6	Given the patient's medication history, do any of the medications increase xerostomia or increase/decrease appetite?	Identify side effects of medications that potentially affect diet	Refer to physician, pharmacist and/or registered dietitian to address issue.
7	Have you lost or gained more than 10 pounds without intending to during the past 6 months?	Unintentional weight loss/gain is an indication of systemic disease	Refer to physician for follow-up

to caries risk might provide additional rationale for behavioral change. Following dietary screening and assessment, food choices and eating behaviors of concern should be identified. The patient's interest in bettering his or her oral and/or systemic health and motivation for behavior change should also be assessed.

Ideally, the clinician negotiates strategies for changes in food choices and/or eating behaviors with the patient; compliance depends on patient investment. Several strategies to achieve behavioral change targeting high-priority needs should be presented to the patient, with the patient choosing how to proceed. Examples of strategies to reduce sugar-sweetened beverage (SSB) intakes are presented in **Table 4** with age-appropriate recommendations for SSB intakes presented in **Table 5**. Although some strategies might take longer than others to achieve the desired change, achievement of change is most important in the long run.

Providing anticipatory guidance to parents of young children as they move throughout childhood is appropriate to prevent development of diet-related caries risk factors. Because toddlers and young children often exert their independence in an effort to obtain preferred foods, parents require support and tools to ensure that they regularly offer appropriate food choices at regular intervals as opposed to ultra-processed foods on demand. Ellyn Satter defines the division of responsibility in feeding in her text, "How to get your child to eat...but not too much" as:

Parents are responsible for what is presented to eat and the manner in which it is presented. Children are responsible for how much and even whether they eat.[15]

Empowering parents with the knowledge and ability to provide both an oral and systemically healthy diet is essential.

Anticipatory guidance for adolescents and adults is also important. Given that one does not choose to eat or not eat, but rather chooses what to eat, one has to consider the composition of the replacement food or beverage—relative energy, caffeine, and nutrient content. Furthermore, changing established dietary behaviors is difficult; provision of anticipatory guidance will support the patient to make desired changes. Patient's food preferences, cooking skills, and time also affect willingness and ability to

Table 4
Strategies to facilitate changes in food choices and eating behaviors

Behavior	Recommendation		Anticipatory Guidance	
	Strategy	Rationale	Concern	Strategy
Excessive intake of SSBs	Switch to sugar-free (SF) version of same beverage	Decrease in SSB intake if SF version accepted	Energy intake: SSBs contain about 14 kcal/oz; depending on total SSB intake, a substantial energy reduction might occur with decreased intake	Encourage consumption of minimally processed foods at structured meals and snacks
	Switch to SF version of different brand	Decrease SSB intake; a different brand might be more acceptable as taste expectations change with brand change	Caffeine intake: caffeinated SSBs may provide significant caffeine intake throughout the day	Encourage gradual reduction of SSB intake, or replacement with caffeinated SF version or alternative caffeine source to reduce headaches and improve likelihood of compliance
	Decrease SSB intake by mixing SSB and SF versions of beverage until SF version is accepted	Gradual change might be more acceptable over time		
	Limit SSB intake to meals	Preferable to prolonged exposure		

Excessive intakes of ultraprocessed foods	Replace ultraprocessed foods with minimally processed foods, balanced according to ChooseMyPlate recommendations	Reduction of added sugars and increased nutrient density for oral and systemic health	Limited acceptance of fruits and vegetables	Encourage gradual increase of fruits and vegetables, different varieties of fruits and vegetables, or methods of preparation to increase likelihood of intake. Refer to registered dietitian for dietary counseling
Frequent and/or prolonged eating events	Encourage intake of minimally processed foods from all food groups at 3 structured meals and 2–3 snacks in sufficient intakes to meet energy requirements	Skipping meals can lead to sipping SSB and frequent snacking to address hunger	Individuals with restrictive eating habits	Refer to registered dietitian for guidance about normal eating; often individuals need permission to consume adequate energy
		Consuming adequate energy at meals and snacks should decrease the desire for lengthy snacking	Individuals with binge eating and/or compulsive overeating behaviors	Refer to physician or registered dietitian for guidance to address eating disorder

From the United States Department of Agriculture. ChooseMyPlate.gov. Available at: https://www.choosemyplate.gov/MyPlate. Accessed 10/3/18.

Table 5
Age-appropriate recommendations for sugar-sweetened beverage intake

Age	Ounces/d	Rationale
0–12 mo	0	SSBs should not replace breast milk, infant formulas, or table foods
1–2 y	0	SSBs should not replace milk and/or table foods
3–5 y	0–4	SSBs are not recommended for preschool children. However, if they are going to be consumed, intakes should be limited. Four ounces (113 g) is consistent with 5% total energy from added sugars
6–12 y	0–6	Six ounces (170 g) is consistent with 5% total energy from added sugars
13–18 y	0–8	Eight ounces (227 g) is consistent with 5% total energy from added sugars
19+ y	0–8	Eight ounces (227 g) is consistent with 5% total energy from added sugars

make changes. Dietary recommendations for food choices and eating behaviors should provide strategies that increase the likelihood of "better" as opposed to "perfect" dietary habits. Anticipatory guidance in dietary changes for diet-related caries risk is provided in **Table 4**.

Patient resources including transportation and buying power affect their ability to comply with recommended changes. Recommendations for changes in food choices and/or eating behaviors must be doable for the patient. Within one's community, knowledge of resources for nutrition education, food resources, and transportation is essential for appropriate referrals. Consultation and collaboration with registered dietitians is recommended for oral health care practitioners whose patient population has significant dietary needs.

SUMMARY

Dental caries is a diet-related disease. Added sugars from ultraprocessed foods, particularly SSBs, are most closely associated with dental caries in observational studies. In addition to added sugar intake, both the frequency and the length of eating events increase caries risk. Oral health care practitioners are responsible for screening every patient for diet-related caries risk factors, and conducting a full assessment with patients identified at risk during screening or having active disease. Effective dietary counseling targets the caries risk behaviors in the context of healthy food choices and dietary behaviors.

REFERENCES

1. United States Department of Health and Human Services and United States Department of Agriculture. 2015-2020 dietary guidelines for Americans. 8th edition. 2015. Available at: https://health.gov/dietaryguidelines/2015/guidelines. Accessed October 10, 2018.
2. United States Department of Agriculture Food and Nutrition Information Center. Dietary reference intakes. Available at: https://www.nal.usda.gov/fnic/dietary-reference-intakes. Accessed October 10, 2018.
3. Food and Nutrition Board, Institute of Medicine, National Academy of Sciences. DRI dietary reference intakes for thiamin, riboflavin, niacin, vitamin B$_6$, folate,

vitamin B_{12}, pantothenic acid, biotin, and choline. Washington, DC: National Academy Press; 1998. Available at: https://www.nap.edu/read/6015/chapter/1. Accessed October 10, 2018.

4. World Health Organization Department of Nutrition for Health and Development. WHO technical information note: sugars and dental caries. 2017. Available at: http://www.who.int/oral_health/publications/sugars-dental-caries-keyfacts/en/. Accessed October 10, 2018.
5. World Health Organization. Guideline: sugars intake for adults and children. Geneva (Switzerland): World Health Organization; 2015. Available at: http://apps.who.int/iris/bitstream/handle/10665/149782/9789241549028_eng.pdf?sequence=1. Accessed October 8, 2018.
6. Marshall TA. Nomenclature, characteristics and dietary intakes of sugars. J Am Dent Assoc 2015;141(1):61–4.
7. United States Food & Drug Administration. Changes to the nutrition facts label. 2018. Available at: https://www.fda.gov/Food/GuidanceRegulation/Guidance DocumentsRegulatoryInformation/LabelingNutrition/ucm385663.htm. Accessed October 9, 2018.
8. Monteiro CA. Invited commentary: nutrition and health: the issue is not food, nor nutrients so much as processing. Public Health Nutr 2009;12(5):729–31.
9. United States Department of Agriculture. ChooseMyPlate. Available at: https://www.choosemyplate.gov/MyPlate. Accessed October 10, 2018.
10. Kral TVE, Chittams J, Moore RH. Relationship between food insecurity, child weight status, and parent-reported child eating and snacking behaviors. J Spec Pediatr Nurs 2017;22(2). https://doi.org/10.1111/jspn.12177.
11. Hammons AJ, Fiese BH. Is frequency of shared family meals related to the nutritional health of children and adolescents? Pediatrics 2011;127(6):1565–74.
12. Brewer JA, Ruf A, Beccia AL, et al. Can mindfulness address maladaptive eating behaviors? Why traditional diet plans fail and how new mechanistic insights may lead to novel interventions. Front Psychol 2018;10(9):1418.
13. Marshall TA. Chairside diet assessment of caries risk. J Am Dent Assoc 2009;140(6):670–4.
14. Juul F, Martinez-Steele E, Parekh N, et al. Ultra-processed food consumption and excess weight among US adults. Br J Nutr 2018;120(1):90–100.
15. Satter E. How to get your kid to eat...but not too much. Palo Alto (CA): Bull Publishing Co; 1987.

Motivational Communication in Dental Practices

Prevention and Management of Caries over the Life Course

Marita R. Inglehart, Dipl. Psych., Dr. phil., Dr. phil. habil.[a,b,*]

KEYWORDS

- Dental caries • Motivational communication • Dentist-patient communication
- Prevention • Pediatric patients • Health education • Dental patients • Life course

KEY POINTS

- Dental practices offer an ideal setting for patient education about the prevention and treatment of oral diseases, specifically dental caries.
- Motivational communication to change patient oral health–related behavior points to the significance of content and process considerations when engaging patients in behavior change communication.
- Content considerations focus on identifying high-priority behavior for change, exploring the patients' affect, behavior, and cognition related to this change, and understanding in which stage of change the patient is.
- The motivational interviewing approach postulates that having empathy, creating a discrepancy in patients' thinking, rolling with resistance to change, and increasing self-efficacy are crucial for ensuring behavior change.
- The motivational communication approach is then used when considering oral health–related behavior change over the life course.

INTRODUCTION

The 2 most common oral diseases—dental caries and periodontitis—are largely preventable. Nevertheless, they remain prevalent even in the United States. For example, in 2017, Dye and colleagues[1] showed that in the United States, 14% of

Disclosure Statement: The author has no relationship with a commercial company that has a direct financial interest in the subject matter or materials discussed in the article or with a company making a competing product.

[a] Department of Periodontics and Oral Medicine, University of Michigan, School of Dentistry, 1011 North University, Ann Arbor, MI 48109-1078, USA; [b] Department of Psychology, College of Literature, Science and Arts (LS&A), University of Michigan, Ann Arbor, MI, USA
* Department of Periodontics and Oral Medicine, University of Michigan, School of Dentistry, 1011 North University, Ann Arbor, MI 48109-1078.
E-mail address: mri@umich.edu

2- to 8-year-old children had untreated dental caries in primary teeth and that the prevalence of caries in older children and adolescents was even higher. In 2018, Eke and colleagues[2] found that 42% of dentate adults 30 years of age or older had periodontitis. Most recently in 2019, Dye and colleagues[3] reported that 11% of adults 50 years or older were edentulous. These statistics come to life when the consequences of having these poor oral health conditions are considered. Research shows that poor oral health affects children's future oral health,[4] their general health,[5,6] quality of life,[7,8] school attendance,[9] and the use of emergency services.[10] Negative effects of adults' poor oral periodontal health on these patients' cardiovascular health,[11] preterm deliveries,[12] and quality of life[13] are also well-documented. The central question clearly is how oral disease in children and adults, and specifically dental caries, can be prevented and how oral health can be improved.

This article makes the argument that dental offices are uniquely well-qualified as settings for initiating successful oral health-related behavior change when engaging patients in motivational communication.

DENTAL OFFICES: A UNIQUE SETTING FOR SUCCESSFUL ORAL HEALTH-RELATED BEHAVIOR CHANGE

In the 1940s and 1950s, researchers at Yale University engaged in an impressive research project aimed at understanding which communication would result in optimal persuasion and ultimate behavior change.[14] Specifically, they analyzed the factors involved in successful communication, namely who should say what to whom, why and when? Their findings showed that the source of a communication—who—should be credible and trustworthy.[15] Dentists are experts in their offices and therefore quite credible as communicators. One example of findings related to the message—what—is the result that a message should focus on one aspect of change and should not try to address too many aspects at one time.[14] In a dental office, a focus on one aspect of behavior, for example, on tobacco cessation counseling or oral hygiene instructions, makes sense owing to the limited time available. Concerning how communication should be presented, Hovland and colleagues found that face-to-face communication is rather successful. Patient–dentist interactions in the dental setting are routinely face-to-face and therefore offer a great setting for behavior change interventions. In summary, dental offices are indeed an excellent setting for communication about oral health behavior change. With this perspective in mind, the question then is why progress in assuring constructive oral health-related behavior is not ideal. The purpose of this article is to analyze which changes in oral health-related communication are needed to successfully engage dental patients in behavior change efforts and to provide examples of specific communication issues over the course of life.

THREE CHALLENGES WHEN COMMUNICATING ABOUT ORAL HEALTH-RELATED BEHAVIOR CHANGE IN DENTAL OFFICES

Systematic reviews showed that there are relationships between tooth brushing frequency and gingival recession,[16] head and neck cancer,[17] periodontitis,[18] and incident and increment of dental caries.[19] However, Rosania and colleagues[20] found that 56% of adults neglect regular brushing and flossing when they are under stress. The relationship between diet, nutrition, and oral health has also been explored extensively[21] and the many ways in which oral health is affected by diet and nutrition are well-documented. Nevertheless, diet-related behavior of the US population is not ideal. The question therefore arises why such large percentages of the US population still suffer from oral diseases that could be largely prevented with oral health promotion efforts.

Three factors might be relevant here. First, it seems that a one-shot approach to health behavior change interactions is frequently taken in dental offices. A problematic behavior is identified and the dentist/dental hygienist engages with the patient in a one-time communication about the problem. We argue that, instead of this one-shot approach, a story line approach over several appointments might result in better outcomes over time.

Second, if an approach is general and not tailored specifically toward a patient, it is rather likely to fail. Instead, using a patent-specific approach by informing a patient why an oral health education is provided based on the findings from their own medical and dental history, their oral examination and radiographs can create interest and open the door to a successful communication. Third, therapeutic interventions aimed at changing behavior such as drug addiction and alcoholism have developed successful process-based approaches to behavior change.[22] We suggest using these approaches to become more successful in creating the basis for successful communication with patients about behavior change.

MOTIVATIONAL COMMUNICATION IN DENTAL PRACTICES: CONTENT AND PROCESS

To move from a one-shot approach to a story line approach, and from a general approach to a patient-centered, tailored approach that uses well-established health behavior change principles from other disciplines, we suggest to engage in motivational communication in dental practices that focuses first on the content of the communication—the what—and then on the process of change—the how.

Motivational Communication: Content Considerations

Three content considerations are important.

- In a first step, it is crucial to identify which specific behavior will be targeted for the change intervention.
- Step 2 focuses on understanding the affective, behavioral, and cognitive (A–B–C) status quo of the patient. How does the patient feel about the behavior change? What are the patient's skills to engage in the behavior and/or which previous behaviors did the patient engage in? What does the patient know and believe about the behavior change? Once we know the A–B–Cs, we can tailor the communication to the patient's situation.
- The third step is to understand at which stage of change the patient is and to realize that we cannot move a patient who is not at all interested in flossing, for example, to flossing regularly in 1 short segment of a dental appointment.

Step 1: Which Behavior Change has the Top Priority for a Specific Patient?

Deciding which specific behavior should be targeted for an educational intervention is exactly like making a treatment plan for a patient. Both are based on the information dentists collected in the medical and dental history, an oral examination, or from radiographs or other sources. Deciding on the content of an educational intervention aimed at increasing patients' oral health promotion efforts uses this information to identify which behavior change is a top priority for this particular patient. A patient's oral health is affected by a multitude of behaviors such as by tooth brushing or flossing, by life style-related behaviors such as using tobacco products or having a high sugar diet, and by general health-related factors such as taking medication that results in xerostomia. Identifying which specific behavior change might be most important is crucial, because trying to change more than one behavior at a time is not likely to succeed.[14,23]

Once a behavior has been identified as the target for a behavior change intervention, the next step is to explore the patient's considerations related to this particular behavior change.

Step 2: Exploring Patients' Affect, Behavior and Cognition: Understanding the A-B-Cs

Patients' considerations concerning their oral health can be categorized as being related to their affective (A), behavioral (B) and cognitive (C) responses to the targeted behavior. Inglehart and Tedesco[24] developed these considerations based on analyzing behavior change approaches in public health, education, and social psychology. **Fig. 1** provides an overview of these 3 components that they summarized as the New Century Model of Oral Health Promotion.

Affective factors are concerned with how patients feel about the behavior they should change, how important it is to them, and how motivated they are to engage in constructive oral health promotion. Their responses differ in the intensity of their affects, but also in the reasons for these responses. For example, patients might refer to esthetic aspects such as "My teeth give me the nicest smile!", or functionality such as "My teeth are great. I can eat and bite everything I want," or their responses can be related to pain or discomfort caused by their teeth. Understanding the content and the intensity of these affective factors is crucial when planning how to motivate a person to change a specific oral health-related behavior.

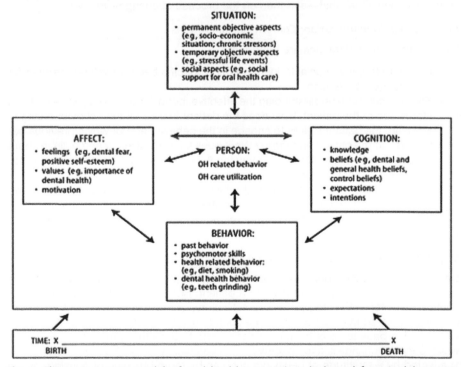

Fig. 1. The new century model of oral health promotion. (*Adapted from* Inglehart MR, Tedesco LA. Behavioral research related to oral hygiene practices: a new century model of oral health promotion. Periodontology 2000 1995;8:15-23; with permission.)

Behavioral factors constitute a second group of patient related factors that need to be understood if behavior change should be successful. Important considerations are to explore whether a patient ever engaged in a certain behavior in the past or if a patient has the skills to engage in a behavior. For example, patients with severe arthritis in their hands will need a distinctly different behavior change approach to assuring good oral hygiene than patients with excellent manual skills.

Cognitions such as health beliefs,[25-27] attitudes, and intentions,[28] as well as patient knowledge about oral health-related matters determine a patient's responses in a conversation. Understanding the patient's perspective and background concerning the targeted behavior is important when determining how to communicate with this patient and which information to introduce.

After a dentist or dental hygienist decides first which behavior has the highest priority for change and second understands the patients' A–B–C considerations in this context, the next step is to explore at which stage of change the patient is.

Step 3: Determining the Patient's Status Quo / Stage of Change

The question at which stage of change a patient is helps to see behavior change from a story line perspective. Prochaska and DiClemente's[29-31] trans theoretic theory offers an insightful and very useful approach to conceptualizing the stages of change as the stages of precontemplation, contemplation, preparation, action, and maintenance. Applying their theory to oral health-related behavior, one could consider a patient in the first stage of precontemplation as not thinking about stopping to smoke or beginning to floss. Moving the patient from this stage to stage 2, the stage of contemplation is therefore crucial. In this stage, patients are aware that a problem exists and are contemplating how they could solve this problem. When patients get ready for change, they move into stage 3, the stage of preparation. They have an intention to change their behavior and begin to make small changes. Stage 4 is the stage of action, in which patients actually show the targeted behavior. They might begin to floss or discontinue drinking sugary drinks. Once patients have reliably established the new behavior, they are in the final stage, the maintenance stage. In this stage, the patients have shown the targeted behavior consistently over a longer period of time. Even in this final stage of change, dental providers should realize that their behavior change work is not done, because their patients might relapse into old behavior patterns.[32] Continuing to positively reinforce the constructive behavior is therefore crucial.

In summary, realizing that change is slow and moves gradually from stage to stage can help providers not to have unrealistic expectations for change. It will help them to see change is an ongoing story and not a one-shot event. After clarifying the content of behavior change by identifying the behavior that is most important to be changed (step 1), getting to know the patient's A–B–C considerations (step 2), and identifying the stage of change a patient is in (step 3), the next question is concerned with the process of change and how change can most likely be achieved. Miller and Rollnick's[22] motivational interviewing (MI) theory is an incredibly helpful approach to engaging more successfully in behavior change efforts.

Motivational Communication: Process Considerations

The importance of the 4 principles of motivational interviewing (MI)
Miller and Rollnick developed the motivational interviewing approach originally to address the change of addictive behavior.[22] Since 2003, research has focused on how MI can be used in dental health care settings to change dental patients' smoking behavior[33-37] or how to change patients' behavior to increase oral health promotion and prevent oral diseases.[38-42]

Central components of MI are the 4 principles that are essential for inducing successful behavior change. The first principle is that the provider needs to show empathy for the client as a starting point of MI.[22] Empathy can be communicated both nonverbally as well as verbally. Nonverbal cues can be, for example, nodding in agreement; verbally communicating empathy can range from sharing own personal experiences to sharing information about other person's similar experiences or statistical supportive information.

The second principle is referred to as creating a discrepancy in the client's mind. When a dentist creates a discrepancy in a patient's mind between the present status (eg, "I do not floss") and the targeted goal (eg, "I should floss daily to prevent periodontal disease"), this discrepancy creates the motivation that fuels the change. Miller and Rollnick[43] therefore stated explicitly "no discrepancy, no motivation"—and thus no change.

As a third principle, they postulated that a provider should "roll with resistance." This principle is concerned with the fact that patients are likely to resist change and that the provider's rolling with the patient's resistance will be crucial to diffusing this negative energy and thus allowing the patient to reflect on the possible potential that a behavior change might have for their lives. The following scenario illustrates this principle. A dentist communicates with a mother of an infant about not putting the infant to bed with a bottle to prevent baby bottle tooth decay. In this situation, some mothers might resist and argue that unless they put their baby to bed with a bottle, the baby will not sleep and the mother will not have any time to rest. Rolling with resistance implies that the dentist communicates understanding for this dilemma and avoids insisting on his point of view and pushing his agenda directly. Instead, the dentist could then carefully explore how the mother would feel about very gradually—over the next 2 to 3 weeks—replacing the cariogenic fluid in the bottle with water by starting out with just a small water replacement and increasing the percentage of water every day a little more until finally the bottle only contains water.

The final principle is related to increasing a sense of self-efficacy in the client. This sense of self-efficacy is an internal awareness that assures the patient that he or she is able to successfully engage in a certain behavior and thus sets the stage to actually perform the behavior. For example, if a patient tells the provider "I cannot floss," this statement signals that the person has a minimal sense of self-efficacy. Unless the provider supports the patient and turns this lack of self-efficacy into a positive sense of self-efficacy, this patient is not likely to engage in flossing behavior. (For a more detailed outline of the application of these 4 principles to oral health-related behavior change, see Inglehart in press.)[44]

The 4 tools: open-ended questions, being affirmative, reflective, and summarizing

In addition to introducing the 4 principles of showing empathy, creating discrepancy, rolling with resistance and increasing self-efficacy, Miller and Rollnick[43] also described 4 tools for creating behavior change. The acronym the authors used for these core interviewing skills is O–A–R–S, which stands for asking open-ended questions, being affirmative, being reflective, and summarizing.

- Asking open-ended questions is like opening a door for the client, giving the client time to think and consider the answer. In some way, open-ended questions provide an opportunity for the dentist to learn something new from the patient.
- Being affirmative instead of critical or judgmental is one way to create a humanistic environment that allows the patient to open up and consider change.
- Reflective responding to a client's statement can offer an opportunity to find out if the client's perspective is accurately perceived. It also communicates to the patient that the provider is trying to understand the patient's point of view.

- Summarizing what was communicated at the end of a communication ensures that patient and dentist are on the same page; they have the same understanding and expectations of the situation.

In summary, combining the content considerations described with the process considerations offered by Miller and Rollnick's MI approach is referred to as motivational communication. **Fig. 2** provides an overview of this motivational communication approach. In motivational communication when changing behavior over the life course, the motivational communication approach is now complemented by specific considerations needed to effectively engage in oral health-related behavior change at different points in life.

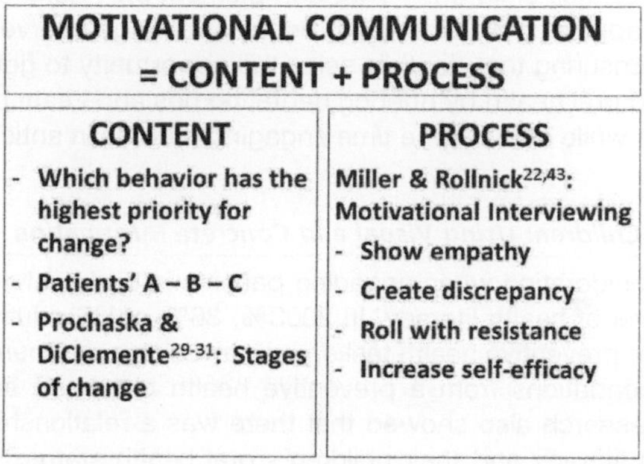

MOTIVATIONAL COMMUNICATION = CONTENT + PROCESS	
CONTENT	**PROCESS**
- Which behavior has the highest priority for change? - Patients' A – B – C - Prochaska & DiClemente[29-31]: Stages of change	Miller & Rollnick[22,43]: Motivational Interviewing - Show empathy - Create discrepancy - Roll with resistance - Increase self-efficacy

Fig. 2. The motivational communication approach.

MOTIVATIONAL COMMUNICATION WHEN CHANGING BEHAVIOR OVER THE LIFE COURSE
Motivational Communication When Providing Behavior Change Education for Different Groups of Patients

When Inglehart and Tedesco[24] introduced their New Century Model of Oral Health Promotion, they also pointed out that oral health promotion efforts have to consider the time in a patient's life at which the oral behavior change occurs (see **Fig. 1**). A discussion of the role of the specific concerns and patient needs in different stages in life on oral health behavior change complements the general motivational communication considerations.

Infant Oral Health Examinations: Anticipatory Guidance and the Power of Establishing a Dental Home

The first ever US Surgeon General Report on Oral Health in 2000 drew attention to the fact that dental caries was the most common chronic childhood disease.[45] Ensuring that parents engage in preventive oral health promotion from early in their child's life has been a goal of the American Academy of Pediatric Dentistry since 1986, when this organization adopted a policy on infant oral health care as a way to promote oral health and prevent oral disease in these very young children.[46] Most recently in 2016, the American Academy of Pediatric Dentistry revisited this guideline on infant oral health care and again stressed the importance of establishing a dental home for infants at the latest by their first birthday.[47]

Once an infant has a dental home, the American Academy of Pediatric Dentistry recommended that a first visit should include taking the infant's medical/dental history and the parent's dental history, conduct an oral examination, demonstrate age-appropriate tooth brushing, assess the infant's risk of developing caries, and determine a prevention plan.[47] In addition, it should focus on providing anticipatory guidance for the parent. The content of this communication should include information for the parent about their infant's dental and oral development, the role of fluoride for the prevention of oral disease, nonnutritive sucking habits, teething, injury prevention, oral hygiene instruction, and the effects of diet on their infant's dentition.[47]

These recommendations point to the important role that families play in oral health promotion for their children.[48] They complement providers' content considerations when they approach an oral health behavior change intervention for parents and their infants. Ensuring that dentists seize the opportunity to get infants off to an early start for good oral health by offering dental homes and infant oral health examinations for infants while at the same time engaging parents in anticipatory guidance is crucial.

Parents of Young Children: Using Visual and Concrete Information

One important consideration when engaging patients in oral health-related behavior change is their level of health literacy. In 2003%, 36% of US adults were unable to perform basic child preventive health tasks, such as using an immunization schedule, following recommendations from a preventive health brochure, and interpreting a growth chart.[49] Research also showed that there was a relationship between caregivers' oral health literacy and their children's oral health status,[50] and that adults with lower oral health literacy were less likely to seek dental care for their children.[51] Additionally, even if parents sought oral health care for their child, the information they received during this visit did not necessarily affect their oral health-related attitudes and behaviors.[52] Benitez and colleagues[53] showed, for example, that informing parents in conversations about putting their child to sleep with a bottle containing juice can cause early childhood caries did not successfully affect this behavior. Despite this evidence, dental providers often rely solely on verbal communication to educate parents about oral health promotion for their child.

One alternative to verbal communication could be to use visual information. Using illustrations when conveying information is supported by research that showed that humans have a preference for picture based, rather than text based information.[54] In addition to using general illustrations in patient education, research also showed that individualizing patient instruction was more effective.[55] Wang and colleagues[56] therefore explored the effects of educating parents of young children in the dental office about their child's upcoming operative appointment by using standardized and/or individualized illustrations or a traditional verbal approach. The standardized visual information consisted of a flip chart that showed pictures of healthy primary teeth versus teeth with different oral health problems. Individualized visual information was provided on an odontogram of primary teeth. Dental hygienists used a green marker to indicate on this chart which dental care the child had received at a visit and used a red marker to circle which dental care was still needed at a next operative visit. The results showed that 46.9% of verbally informed parents missed the next operative appointment compared with only 19.1% of parents who had received information with the help of standardized illustrations, 15.6% who had received individualized illustrations, and 10.4% who had received both individualized and standardized visual information. A follow-up study by Picard and colleagues[57] showed that educating parents with visual aids versus verbally after their child's treatment under general anesthesia improved their attendance at follow-up appointments significantly.

In summary, using individualized and standardized illustrations for oral health education about oral health promotion can complement motivational communication efforts and clearly increases the effectiveness of these educational interventions.

Oral Health Education for 5- to 10-Year-Old Children: The Benefits of Experiential Learning

Although visual information has been shown to be effective in health education change efforts with parents, experiential learning can be a successful way to educate children as young as 5 years of age. Developmental psychology showed that children in this age group are likely to benefit from hands-on, experiential learning.[58] The question is whether experiential learning can be successfully used with children in dental offices. Inglehart and colleagues[59] tested the effectiveness of an experiential approach to educating Kindergarten and elementary school age children in a dental office. They found that children with experiential educational experiences in a dental office were more likely to brush their teeth on their own, to provide oral health-related reasons for brushing, to floss their teeth, and to floss more frequently and by themselves than children before the experiential intervention and children who had received traditional verbal oral health education. A 2-week follow-up phone call with the parents of children in the experiential group provided further evidence for the positive effects of practice-based experiential oral hygiene-related instruction for young children and even for their parents. Future research should explore how these experiential efforts can be introduced more widely.

Adolescence: A Time of Change and Risks

Adolescent patients have distinctive characteristics and needs.[60,61] They have high caries rates,[1,60,62] an increased risk for traumatic injuries,[60] a tendency for poor nutritional habits[60] such as drinking excessive amounts of soft drinks,[63] an increased interest in appearance-related aesthetics,[64] high rates of dental phobia,[42,65,66] and special social and psychological needs.[60] At the same time, research found a deterioration of oral hygiene efforts during this time. Given that adolescence also is a time when life style related habits might be created such as smoking, it is clearly important to identify new ways to educate adolescents about oral health-related issues should be explored. Using visual information might be one way to more successfully educate pediatric patients in this age group.[62] Motivational communication efforts must consider the unique characteristics and needs of this age group.

Oral Health Behavior Change and Adults: Addressing Destructive Habits and Educating the Educators

When considering oral health behavior change in adults, 2 central areas are of concern. The first area is the way motivational communication could be used to change destructive life style related behaviors such as smoking or chewing tobacco, and diet-related behavior such as the consumption of foods and beverages with high sugar content.

The second area of concern focuses on the relationship between oral health and systemic health such as diabetes[67] and mental health such as eating disorders[68] or depression.[69]

Although the relationships between, for example, periodontal disease and diabetes are widely discussed, considering the role of dental care providers in engaging patients with mental health issues in constructive oral health promotion efforts receives much less attention. This situation is unfortunate because mental health issues such as addictions, anxiety disorders and affective disorders are prevalent in the United States[70] and can have a significant effect on patients' oral health and oral health care use. In addition, medications for mental health issues are likely to cause xerostomia, which further compromises patients' oral health. More research is needed to assure that educational efforts will be developed for dental care providers to realize the crucial role they can play in promoting good oral health among patients with mental health concerns.

In addition to these 2 main considerations, the fact that the percentage of older adults over 65 years of age in the US is rapidly increasing should draw attention to the importance of considering how motivational communication can be optimally used with this patient population. Gaining a better understanding of the ways in which motivational communication with adults over 65 years of age are affected by age related changes is therefore crucial. For example, understanding how sensory and cognitive changes related to aging affect communication in dental offices and beyond is crucial when engaging in motivational communication.[71,72] These communication efforts become especially challenging when communicating with patients with mild, moderate or severe neurocognitive deficits previously referred to as dementia[73] or patients who have been recently bereaved or face death.[74,75]

SUMMARY AND OUTLOOK

This article offered a new approach called Motivational Communication as a way to structure oral health-related patient education and then considered how each stage in life adds specific considerations in this context. A need for more research in this field became obvious when taking this life course approach. Three additional areas that have so far been neglected come to mind.

- First, social and cultural influences, such as unconscious biases,[76] are likely to affect our communication about oral health behavior change. More research is needed to understand how these processes can affect communication with patients from different socioeconomic and/or ethnic/racial backgrounds, with different gender identities or sexual orientations, with different abilities or from different religious backgrounds—to name just a few of the many social identities that patients have. Research about cross-cultural communication issues and communication breakdowns in dental offices are clearly needed to raise dental care providers' awareness concerning these issues.
- Second, time and financial constraints limit the efforts that dentists and even dental hygienists can devote to oral health behavior change in one-on-one settings. Taking oral health education to the communities such as to Head Start programs, Kindergarten classes and other schools as well as to community groups with adults and to residential homes for older adults and nursing homes is clearly important. A comprehensive motivational communication approach for community-based education is needed.
- Third, deliberate efforts to connect motivational communication efforts with preventive dentistry strategies such as fluoride applications and the use of dental sealants and other preventive treatments are crucial and need to be developed in the future. Training dental care providers to use a motivational communication when explaining the benefits of these approaches could increase acceptance.

REFERENCES

1. Dye BA, Mitnik GL, Iafolla TJ, et al. Trends in dental caries in children and adolescents according to poverty status in the United States from 1999 through 2004 and from 2011 through 2014. J Am Dent Assoc 2017;148(8):550–65.e7.

2. Eke PI, Thornton-Evans GO, Wei L, et al. Periodontitis in US adults: National Health and Nutrition Examination Survey 2009-2014. J Am Dent Assoc 2018; 149(7):576–88.e6.
3. Dye BA, Weatherspoon DJ, Lopez Mitnik G. Tooth loss among older adults according to poverty status in the United States from 1999 through 2004 and 2009 through 2014. J Am Dent Assoc 2019;150(1):9–23.e3.
4. Greenwall AL, Johnsen D, DiSantis TA, et al. Longitudinal evaluation of caries patterns from the primary to the mixed dentition. Pediatr Dent 1990;12:278–82.
5. Ayhan H, Suskan E, Yildirim S. The effect of nursing or rampant caries on height, body weight and head circumference. J Clin Pediatr Dent 1996;20:209–12.
6. van Gemert-Schriks MCM, van Amerongen EW, Aartman IHA, et al. The influence of dental caries on body growth in prepubertal children. Clin Oral Investig 2011; 15:141–9.
7. Inglehart MR, Filstrup SL, Wandera A. Oral health related quality of life and children. In: Inglehart MR, Bagramian RA, editors. Oral health and quality of life. Chicago: Quintessence Publ. Company; 2002 [Chapter: 8].
8. Filstrup SL, Briskie D, da Fonseca M, et al. Early childhood caries and quality of life – child and parent perspectives. Pediatr Dent 2003;25(5):431–40.
9. Gift HC, Reisine ST, Larach DC. The social impact of dental problems and visits. Am J Public Health 1992;82(12):1663–8.
10. Sheller B, Williams BJ, Lombardi SM. Diagnosis and treatment of dental caries-related emergencies in a children's hospital. Pediatr Dent 1997;19(8):470–5.
11. Genco R, Offenbacher S, Beck S. Periodontal disease and cardiovascular disease: epidemiology and possible mechanisms. J Am Dent Assoc 2002; 133(Suppl):14S–22S.
12. Offenbacher S, Boggess KA, Murtha AP, et al. Progressive periodontal disease and risk of very preterm delivery. Obstet Gynecol 2006;107(1):29–36.
13. Inglehart MR, Bagramian RA, editors. Oral health and quality of life. Chicago: Quintessence Publ. Company; 2002.
14. Hovland CI, Janis IL, Kelley HH. Communication and persuasion: psychological studies of opinion change. New Haven (CT): Yale University Press; 1953.
15. Hovland CI, Weiss W. Influence of source credibility on communication effectiveness. Public Opin Q 1951;15(4):635–50.
16. Rajapakse PS, McCracken GI, Gwynnett E, et al. Does tooth brushing influence the development and progression of non-inflammatory gingival recession? A systematic review. J Clin Periodontol 2007;34(12):1046–61.
17. Zeng XT, Leng WD, Zhang C, et al. Meta-analysis on the association between tooth brushing and head and neck cancer. Oral Oncol 2015;51(5):446–51.
18. Zimmermann H, Zimmermann N, Hagenfeld D, et al. Is frequency of tooth brushing a risk factor for periodontitis? A systematic review and meta-analysis. Community Dent Oral Epidemiol 2015;43(2):116–27.
19. Kumar S, Tadakamadla J, Johnson NW. Effect of tooth brushing frequency on incidence and increment of dental caries: a systematic review and meta-analysis. J Dent Res 2016;95(11):1230–6.
20. Rosania AE, Low KG, McCormick CM, et al. Stress, depression, cortisol, and periodontal disease. J Periodontol 2009;80(2):260–6.
21. Palmer CA, Boyd LD. Diet and nutrition in oral health. 3rd edition. New York: Pearson; 2017.
22. Miller WR, Rollnick S. Motivational interviewing: helping people change. 3rd edition. New York: Guilford Press; 2013.

23. McGuire WJ. The Yale communication and attitude change program in the 1950s. In: Dennis EE, Wartella EA, editors. American communication research: the remembered history. Mahwah (NJ): Lawrence Erlbaum Associates; 1996. p. 39–59 [Chapter 3].

24. Inglehart MR, Tedesco LA. Behavioral research related to oral hygiene practices: a new century model of oral health promotion. Periodontol 2000 1995;8:15–23.

25. Becker MH, editor. The health belief model and personal health behavior, vol. 2. Health Education Monographs; 1974. p. 324–473.

26. Becker MH. Understanding patient compliance: the contributions of attitudes and other psychosocial factors. In: Cohen SJ, editor. New directions in patient compliance. Lexington (MA): Health; 1979.

27. Becker MH, Rosenstock IM. Compliance with medical advice. In: Steptoe A, Mathews A, editors. Health care and human behavior. London: Academic Press; 1984.

28. Fishbein M, Ajzen I. Attitudes towards toward objects as predictors of single and multiple behavioral criteria. Psychol Rev 1974;81(1):59–74.

29. Prochaska JO, DiClemente CC. Stages and processes of self-change in smoking: toward an integrative model of change. J Consult Clin Psychol 1983;51(3): 390–5.

30. Prochaska JO, DiClemente CC. The transtheoretical approach: crossing traditional boundaries of change. Homewood (IL): Dorsey Press; 1984.

31. Prochaska JO, DiClemente CC, Norcross JC. In search of how people change: applications to addictive behaviors. Am Psychol 1992;47(9):1102–14.

32. Marlatt GA, Gordon JR. Theoretical rationale and overview of the model. In: Marlatt GA, Gordon JR, editors. Relapse prevention: maintenance strategies in addictive behavior change. New York: The Guilford Press; 1985. p. 3–70.

33. Davis JM, Stockdale MS, Cropper M. The need for tobacco education: studies of collegiate dental hygiene patients and faculty. J Dent Educ 2005;69(12):1340–52.

34. Ramseier CA, Mattheos N, Needleman I, et al. Consensus report: First European Workshop on tobacco use prevention and cessation for oral health professionals. Oral Health Prev Dent 2006;4(1):7–18.

35. Ramseier CA, Christen A, McGowan J, et al. Tobacco use prevention and cessation in dental and dental hygiene undergraduate education. Oral Health Prev Dent 2006;4(1):49–60.

36. Ramseier CA, Bornstein MM, Saxer UP, et al. Tobacco use prevention and cessation in the dental practice. Schweizer Monatsschr Zahnmed 2007;117(3):253–78.

37. Koerber A, Crawford J, O'Connell K. The effects of teaching dental students brief motivational interviewing for smoking-cessation counseling: a pilot study. J Dent Educ 2003;67(4):439–47.

38. Weinstein P, Harrison R, Benton T. Motivating parents to prevent caries in their young children: one-year findings. J Am Dent Assoc 2004a;135(6):731–8.

39. Weinstein P, Harrison R, Benton T. Comment in. J Am Dent Assoc 2004;135(9): 1224 [author reply: 2004b; 1224–6; 135(6):731–8].

40. Weinstein P, Harrison R, Benton T. Motivating mothers to prevent caries: confirming the beneficial effect of counseling. J Am Dent Assoc 2006;137(6):789–93.

41. Harrison R, Benton T, Everson-Stewart S, et al. Effect of motivational interviewing on rates of early childhood caries: a randomized trial. Pediatr Dent 2007;29(1): 16–22.

42. Skaret E, Raadal M, Berg E, et al. Dental anxiety and dental avoidance among 12 to 18 year olds in Norway. Eur J Oral Sci 1999;107(6):422–8.

43. Miller WR, Rollnick S. Motivational interviewing: preparing people to change. 2nd edition. New York: Guilford Press; 2002.
44. Inglehart MR. [Chapter: 21]. Oral health behavior change and oral health promotion. In AAPHD: Dentistry, dental practice and the community. 7th edition. Elsevier Inc. Publishing Company, Jan. 2020.
45. United States Department of Health and Human Services. Oral health in America: a report of the surgeon general. Rockville (MD): U.S. Department of Health and Human Services, National Institute of Dental and Craniofacial Research, National Institutes of Health; 2000.
46. American Academy of Pediatric Dentistry. Policy on infant oral health care. Reference Manual 1986;37(6):15–6.
47. American Academy of Pediatric Dentistry. Perinatal and infant oral health care. Reference Manual 2016;40(6):18–9.
48. Inglehart MR, Tedesco LA. The role of the family in preventing oral diseases. In: Cohen LK LK, Gift HC, editors. Disease prevention and oral health promotion - socio-dental sciences in action. Copenhagen (Denmark): Munksgaard; 1995. p. 271–307.
49. Kutner ME, Greenberg E, Jin Y, et al. The health literacy of America's adults: results from the 2003 National Assessment of adult literacy. Washington, DC: National Center for Education Statistics; U.S. Department of Education, National Center for Education Statistics publication 2006-2483; 2006.
50. Bridges SM, Parthasarathy DS, Wong HM, et al. The relationship between caregiver functional oral health literacy and child oral health status. Patient Educ Couns 2014;94(3):411–6.
51. Miller E, Lee JY, DeWalt DA, et al. Impact of caregiver literacy on children's oral health outcomes. Pediatrics 2010;126:107–14.
52. Kanellis MJ, Logan HL, Jakobsen J. Changes in maternal attitude toward baby bottle tooth decay. Pediatr Dent 1997;19(1):56–60.
53. Benitez C, O'Sullivan D, Tinanoff N. Effect of a preventive approach for the treatment of nursing bottle caries. ASDC J Dent Child 1994;61(1):46–9.
54. Sansgiry SS, Cady PS, Adamcik BA. Consumer comprehension of information on over-the-counter medication labels: effects of picture superiority and individual differences based on age. J Pharm Mark Manage 1997;11:63–76.
55. McBride CM, Emmons KM, Lipkus IM. Understanding the potential of teachable moments: the case of smoking cessation. Health Educ Res 2003;18(2):156–70.
56. Wang SJ, Briskie D, Hu J, et al. Illustrated information for parent education - Parent and patient responses. Pediatr Dent 2010;32:295–303.
57. Picard AJ, Estrella MR, Boynton J, et al. Educating parents of children receiving comprehensive dental care under general anesthesia with visual aids. Pediatr Dent 2014;36(4):329–35.
58. Piaget J, Inhelder B. The psychology of the child. 2nd Edition. New York: Basic Books; 1969.
59. Inglehart MR, Maples S, Boynton J, et al. Practice-based experiential oral health education for 5-10 year old children. Fort Lauderdale (FL): American Association of Dental Research Meeting; 2018.
60. American Academy of Pediatric Dentistry. Clinical guidelines on adolescent oral health care. Reference Manual 2009;29(7):07–8.
61. Edelstein BL. Disparities in oral health and access to care: findings of national surveys. Ambul Pediatr 2002;2(2 Suppl):141–7.
62. Ertugrul HZ. Informing adolescent dental patients and their parents about oral health care needs – analyzing the effects of using visual aides [Master's thesis].

Horace H. Rackham School of Graduate Studies, Ann Arbor (MI): The University of Michigan; 2010.

63. Majewski RF. Dental caries in adolescents associated with caffeinated carbonated beverages. Pediatr Dent 2001;23(3):198–203.

64. Brukiene V, Aleksejuniene J. An overview of oral health promotion in adolescents. Int J Paediatr Dent 2009;19:163–71.

65. Skaret E, Raadal M, Berg E, et al. Dental anxiety among 18-year-olds in Norway: prevalence and related factors. Eur J Oral Sci 1998;106(4):835–43.

66. Skaret E, Weinstein P, Kvale G, et al. An intervention program to reduce dental avoidance behaviour among adolescents: a pilot study. Eur J Paediatr Dent 2003;4(4):191–6.

67. Thepwongsa I, Muthukumar R, Kessomboon P. Motivational interviewing by general practitioners for Type 2 diabetes patients: a systematic review. Fam Pract 2017;34(4):376–83.

68. Frimenko KM, Murdoch-Kinch CA, Inglehart MR. Education about eating disorders: dental students' perceptions and practice of interprofessional care. J Dent Educ 2017;81(11):1327–37.

69. McFarland M, Inglehart M. Depression, self-efficacy, and oral health – an exploration. OHDMBSC 2010;9(4):214–22.

70. Black DW, Andreasen NC. Introductory textbook to psychiatry. 6th edition. Washington, DC: American Psychiatric Association Publishing; 2014.

71. Goldblatt RS, Yellowitz JA. The senior friendly office. In: Friedman PK, editor. Geriatric dentistry: caring for our aging population. Hoboken, NJ: John Wiley & Sons; 2014. p. 43–58 [Chapter: 5].

72. Stein PS, Aalboe JA, Savage MW, et al. Strategies for communicating with older dental patients. J Am Dent Assoc 2014;145(2):159–64.

73. Black WD, Andreasen NC. Introductory textbook of psychiatry. 6th edition. Washington, DC: American Psychiatric Publishing; 2014. p. 439–58.

74. Gawande A. Being mortal: medicine and what matters in the end. New York: Metropolitan Books, Henry Holt and Company; 2014.

75. Kessler D. The needs of the dying: a guide for bringing hope, comfort, and love to life's final chapter. New York: Harper Collins Publ; 2000.

76. Devine PG, Forscher PS, Austin AJ, et al. Long-term reduction in implicit race bias: a prejudice habit breaking intervention. J Exp Soc Psychol 2012;48(6): 1267–78.

Personalized Dental Caries Management in Children

Martha Ann Keels, DDS, PhD[a,b,*]

KEYWORDS

- Dental caries • Caries lesion • Children • Primary dentition

KEY POINTS

- Clinicians should be familiar with the 3 main dental caries patterns that occur in the primary dentition—early childhood caries (ECC), late childhood caries (LCC), and primary second molar hypoplasia with carious involvement (PSMH-C).
- ECC is redefined to terminate at age 3 years in order to not overlap with LCC or PSMH-C and more closely match the time period of infant and toddler feeding behaviors.
- LCC develops after the closure of the proximal spaces between the first and second primary molars. This closure of the space between the primary molars occurs approximately at age 4 years, commensurate with the initial emergence of the permanent first molars within the alveolus.
- PSMH-C is recognized immediately after the eruption of the primary second molar and may be the first sign of molar-incisor hypomineralization involving the permanent first molars and permanent maxillary incisors.
- The extent of the caries disease process within each pattern should be considered prior to developing a plan for disease management and a strategy for prevention.

INTRODUCTION

Dental caries in the primary dentition prior to age 6 years is the most common chronic condition among children in the United States.[1] Over the past several decades, dental caries experience in children has focused predominantly on early childhood caries (ECC).[2,3] ECC, formerly known as nursing bottle caries, baby bottle tooth decay, night bottle mouth, and night bottle caries, is defined as a dental disease that affects children between birth and age 6 years. ECC is characterized by the presence of 1 or more decayed (noncavitated or cavitated lesions), missing (due to caries), or filled tooth surfaces in any primary tooth.[4,5] The life cycle of the primary dentition begins to emerge at approximately age 6 months, with the eruption of the mandibular central incisors, and concludes with the exfoliation of the primary maxillary canines at

[a] Department of Pediatric Dentistry, University of North Carolina School of Dentistry, 2711 North Duke Street, Durham, NC 27704, USA; [b] Department of Pediatrics, Duke University, Durham, NC, USA
* Department of Pediatric Dentistry, University of North Carolina School of Dentistry, 2711 North Duke Street, Durham, NC 27704.
E-mail address: marthaann.keels@duke.edu

Dent Clin N Am 63 (2019) 621–629
https://doi.org/10.1016/j.cden.2019.06.002
0011-8532/19/© 2019 Elsevier Inc. All rights reserved.

approximately 12 years of age. There has been little focus on the caries experience in the primary dentition beyond 6 years of age. This article highlights 2 additional dental caries patterns presenting in the primary dentition along with their prevention and management strategies.

REDEFINING CARIES PATTERNS IN THE PRIMARY DENTITION

The classic clinical presentation of ECC early in life involves carious involvement of the 4 maxillary incisors with or without involvement of the first primary molars because these teeth are in the pathway of exposure to sugar-containing liquids, including breastmilk and infant formulas. The position of the tongue while breastfeeding or drinking from a bottle or sippy cup blankets the lower incisors and prevents any sugar-containing liquid from coming into contact with these teeth. This pattern typically presents itself prior to the age of 3 years (Martha Ann Keels, DDS, PhD, Erica A. Brecher, DMD, MS, Unpublished Data, 2019). In other words, from clinical experience, if a child reaches the age of 36 months without experiencing any carious lesions affecting the maxillary incisors, then it is highly unlikely these maxillary anterior teeth will become carious. Another important observation involving the first primary molar in the ECC pattern is that the carious process typically starts on the occlusal surface and can spread laterally onto the mesial and/or distal surfaces. If diagnosed early, then the remaining dentition can be protected as the primary canines and primary second molars erupt after the first molars. In most children, infant and toddler feeding behaviors (eg, breastfeeding or bottle feeding through the night) contributing to ECC have ceased prior to the eruption of the primary canines and second primary molars. Thus, age 3 years is a natural cutoff for redefining ECC, based on the significant contribution of infant and toddler feeding to this disease pattern as well as a child's transition to a school setting at age 4 years.

In a retrospective chart review of 25 years in a private pediatric dental practice in an urban community providing dental care for more than 6000 children ages birth to 21 years (70% with private dental coverage and 30% with Medicaid coverage), 3 distinct dental caries patterns were observed in the primary dentition (Martha Ann Keels, DDS, PhD, Erica A. Brecher, DMD, MS, Unpublished Data, 2019) (**Fig. 1**); 25% of the children had dental caries involving the 4 maxillary incisors with or without involvement of the maxillary first primary molars (**Fig. 2**). All of these children were predominantly under the age of 3 years. The second pattern affecting most of the children was interproximal dental caries involving the distal surface of the first primary molars and the mesial surface of the second primary molars (**Fig. 3**); 70% of the children with dental caries presented with this pattern. The third pattern, which was the least prevalent, occurring less than 5% of the time, was dental caries associated with enamel hypoplasia of the 4 primary second molars (**Fig. 4**). There were some children older than 3 years of age, who had not seen a dentist, who were diagnosed with various combinations of the 4 patterns of dental caries. This article focuses on the predominant 3 patterns observed.

In this private practice setting, the classic presentation of ECC occurred prior to the age of 3 years. A majority of children presenting with LCC had not experienced ECC prior to developing the posterior interproximal disease. For purposes of this article, ECC is redefined to match more closely the disease pattern that it was meant to reflect (nursing bottle caries, baby bottle tooth decay, night bottle mouth, and night bottle caries), thus limiting ECC from birth to the age of 3 years.[6] This revised classification allows for a more precise and targeted approach to disease prevention and management. Having the ECC definition extend beyond age 3 years masks the ability to recognize and study other dental caries patterns occurring in the primary dentition.

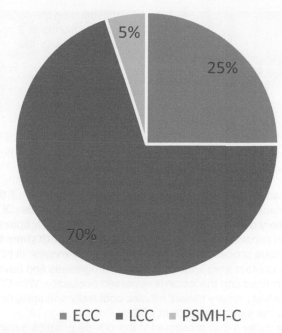

■ ECC ■ LCC ■ PSMH-C

Fig. 1. Primary dental caries patterns.

The most prevalent dental caries pattern in the primary dentition, observed in the private practice setting 70% of the time, initiated after the closure of the proximal contacts between the first and second primary molars. This disease pattern is now referred to as late childhood caries (LCC).[7] There are potentially 8 interproximal lesions that can occur with LCC. The lesions can vary in depth on each surface. It is possible that a practitioner diagnoses LCC with the initial presentation of 1 interproximal surface affected or any combination all the way up to involving all 8 surfaces. The severe form of LCC has, in addition to interproximal caries between the primary molars, dental caries involvement of the mesial of the first primary molars and the distal of the primary canines, resulting in, potentially, 16 interproximal lesions. A child manifesting severe LCC generally is characterized by severe dental crowding and lack of

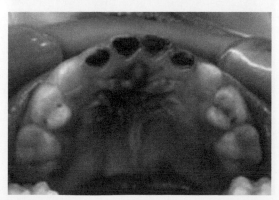

Fig. 2. Example of Classic ECC, where the primary maxillary incisors and first molars are affected.

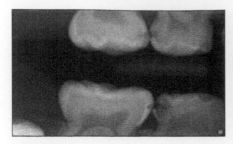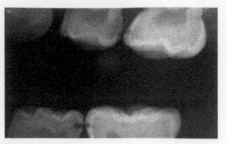

Fig. 3. Right and left bitewing radiographic example of LCC in a 4 year old, where 8 interproximal surfaces are carious. No other lesions were detected.

developmental spacing between the posterior teeth. The timing of the physiologic closure of the contact between the first and second primary molars is approximately age 4 years. A primary dentition that maintains the developmental spacing is less likely to develop LCC. An important observation that distinguishes LCC from ECC is the progression of the carious process involving the first primary molars. In LCC, the carious lesion starts at the contact area and, as the lesion progresses and cavitates, the marginal ridge is undermined and the lesion is visualized occlusally. With ECC, the carious lesion involving the first primary molars initiates occlusally and spreads laterally to the proximal surfaces, the exact opposite of LCC.

The third unique pattern that presented in the private practice setting was carious involvement subsequent to enamel hypoplasia affecting the second primary molars. In most cases, the children with primary second molar hypoplasia (PSMH) had no other dental caries experience. This pattern is apparent after the second primary

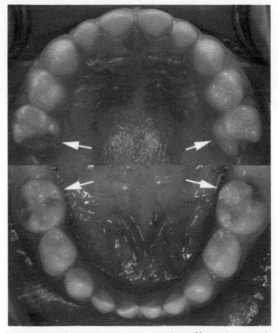

Fig. 4. Example of PSMH-C. The arrows point to the affected second molars. (Copyright © American Academy of Pediatric Dentistry and reproduced with their permission.)

molars emerge through the gingiva at approximately ages 23 months to 33 months. If PSMH has carious involvement it is referred to as PSMH with caries involvement (PSMH-C) versus PSMH with noncarious involvement.

Recognizing which dental caries pattern exists in a child is a first critical step in formulating the best strategy for management of the disease as well as developing the most effective preventive plan.

PREVENTION AND MANAGEMENT OF EARLY CHILDHOOD CARIES

Educating mothers during pregnancy about instituting good oral hygiene routines for themselves and their baby is an important first step in preventing ECC. Having a child's primary medical health care provider encourage good oral health habits and establishing a dental home by age 1 year are also important in the prevention of ECC.[8,9] Good oral health habits include ensuring the caregiver is involved in adequate removal of the oral biofilm twice daily, use of a smear of fluoridated toothpaste (0.1 mg of fluoride) no larger than a grain of rice, and interdental cleaning for any 2 teeth that are touching.[10–13] Dietary counseling regarding the cariogenic risks of frequently consuming liquids and foods high in carbohydrates or acidity should be reviewed with caregivers. The increased caries risk of feeding during the night should also be emphasized. A child's caries risk should be reassessed at least every 6 months to ensure compliance with known preventive measures.[14]

Given that the diagnosis of ECC occurs prior to age 3 years, managing a child's behavior becomes a critical aspect of stabilizing and restoring carious maxillary incisors with or without involvement of the first primary molars. Another factor to take into consideration is the safety of sedation or general anesthesia in a child under 3 years of age. The US Food and Drug Administration issued a warning that repeated or lengthy use of general anesthetic and sedation drugs during procedures in children younger than 3 years may affect the development of children's brains.[15] Consequently, the use of noninvasive techniques to stabilize ECC prior to age 3 is important in delaying dental treatment under sedation or general anesthesia. Both noncavitated lesions and cavitated lesions not encroaching on the pulp can be managed nonsurgically.[16,17] To stabilize the carious lesions, in-office professionally applied fluorides, such as fluoride varnish for noncavitated lesions or silver diamine fluoride (SDF) for cavitated lesions, can be used. The Alternative Restorative Technique also can be used to stabilize cavitated carious lesions. Once a lesion cavitates, then it must be stabilized with a glass inomer cement (GIC), resin-modified glass inomer (RMGI), or composite resin (CR). If the carious lesion has extended beyond the capabilities of the glass inomer (GI) or resins, then full coverage is indicated with either an esthetic resin-veneered stainless steel crown or zirconium crown.[18] If a pulpectomy is indicated, then the medicament of choice is one that easily resorbs with exfoliation, such as zinc oxide and eugenol. If the primary incisor is unrestorable, then extraction is indicated. Space maintenance in the anterior is indicated only if space loss is anticipated with an active digit habit.[19] Detailed evidenced-based strategies for nonsurgical and surgical management of dental caries in the primary dentition are discussed in Margherita Fontana's article, "Nonrestorative Management of Cavitated and Noncavitated Caries Lesions," and Andrea G. Ferreira Zandona's article, "Surgical Management of Caries Lesions: Selective Removal of Carious Tissues," in this iusse.

PREVENTION AND MANAGEMENT OF LATE CHILDHOOD CARIES

Given the presentation of LCC involves initially the proximal surfaces, preventive strategies must target disrupting the biofilm that accumulates in the proximal contact area in addition to the previously described preventive strategies for ECC. The most recognized technique for cleaning the proximal surfaces is dental flossing. Hujoel and coauthors[13] systematically reviewed the effect of flossing on interproximal caries risk in children ages 4 years to 13 years and found that professional flossing on school days was associated with a 40% caries risk reduction. Self-flossing was shown to be not effective in this age group. Therefore, supervised flossing by trained caregivers in children with closed proximal contacts should be recommended.[13] Flossing immediately after the consumption of a tenacious carbohydrate also may be beneficial. Children with posterior interproximal spacing have interproximal surfaces that are naturally more self-cleansing with saliva or water and naturally less prone to interproximal cavitation.

The role of masticated foods in addition to the role of SCL also should be considered in the etiology of LCC. The easier it is for a food or candy to adhere in the proximal area, the harder it is for the food material to disintegrate. The longer a fermentable carbohydrate remains in contact with the proximal tooth surface, the more it increases the risk of dental caries. Clinicians should recommend avoiding sticky or gummy carbohydrates. Treats that melt easily are preferable to ones that are sticky or gummy. Non–sugar-containing and low acidic beverages also should be encouraged to avoid making the biofilm more acidic.

Similar to prevention of ECC, clinicians should recommend brushing at home twice a day with a fluoridate toothpaste in the recommended dosage size by age. For children between the ages of 3 years and 6 years, the amount of fluoridated toothpaste dispensed should be limited to a pea-sized amount (0.25 mg of fluoride) to maximize the caries prevention effect and minimize the risk of fluorosis.[9] Fluoride varnish also should be applied professionally at least twice a year.

Once the interproximal lesions become cavitated, then a nonsurgical approach can be attempted with applications interproximally with fluoride varnish or resin infiltration but carefully monitoring with bitewing radiographs is indicated. Once a lesion progresses radiographically to a stage that suggests likely cavitation, then the lesion must be stabilized with a GIC, resin-modified glass inomer, or composite resin. If the carious lesion has extended beyond the capabilities of the GI or resins, then full coverage is indicated with either a stainless steel crown or zirconium crown.[18] The Hall technique of crown placement may be indicated if managing a child's behavior is difficult.[20,21] If a pulpotomy is indicated, then mineral trioxide aggregate or formocresol should be the medicament of choice based on the 2017 systematic review by Coll and others.[22] Pulpectomies are an option for nonvital second primary molars. The medicament of choice is one that easily resorbs with exfoliation, such as zinc oxide and eugenol. If the primary molar is unrestorable, then extraction is indicated followed by placing the appropriate space maintainer (eg, distal shoe or band and loop), because it is critical to maintain the mesial-distal width of the carious teeth in order to preserve natural arch form and minimize dental crowding.[19]

After the closure of the proximal spaces between the primary molars in all 4 quadrants, the clinician should obtain bitewing radiographs to visualize the health of the posterior interproximal surfaces. Given that LCC can involve 8 surfaces and severe LCC may involve 16 surfaces, it is incumbent on the clinician to be looking for this pattern and not focus on just 1 clinically carious molar. Seeing that a child has all 4 quadrants involved, then a discussion should follow on how to best manage LCC and protect the child's developing psyche. With the more anxious child, it may be more prudent to restore these 8 interproximal lesions in 1 appointment under general anesthesia versus several individual appointments. If restoring 1 quadrant at a time is attempted in an outpatient clinical setting, then the child's opinion of the first procedure must be taken into account. It is not uncommon for a child to develop an opinion of the treatment process and then subsequently dread future appointments. The effort to restore the remaining quadrants may become more challenging and potentially contribute to form-ing a dentally resistant and phobic patient. Every effort should be taken to help alleviate the child's anxiety and maintain the child's trust throughout the restorative care.

PREVENTION AND MANAGEMENT OF HYPOPLASTIC SECOND PRIMARY MOLARS

Given that the etiology of PSMH is not completely elucidated, it is difficult to success-fully prevent the hypoplastic event. Studies to date examining the etiology of molar-incisor hypomineralization (MIH) in permanent dentition have pinpointed prolonged infections during the mineralization stage. Questions remain as to whether it is the febrile state associated with the illness or the antibiotics used to treat the illness. It is important for the medical community to manage an infection judiciously and reduce the fever as quickly as possible to potentially reduce the risk of formation of hypoplastic molars. Once these teeth emerge into the oral cavity at approximately 28 months, it is critical to make the caregiver aware of the increased risk of dental caries. In the dental office, professionally applied topical fluoride varnish is indicated until a more definitive restorative plan can be rendered.[16] If the molars are hypersensitive, then an application of SDF is indicated. Multiple applications may be necessary to reduce the sensitivity. SDF should not be used if there is concomitant caries approaching the pulpal tissue.[16] Depending on the amount of tooth structure affected, the clinician may need to smooth the rough edges of the affected molars for comfort as well as create a more self-cleansable surface by applying a restorative material, such as a sealant, GIC, compos-ite resin, stainless steel crown, or zirconium crown.[18] The selection of the restorative method should be based on the amount of sound tooth structure remaining. If the pri-mary molar is nonrestorable, then dental extraction is indicated and the appropriate space maintainer placed to prevent mesial drift of the permanent first molars.[19]

RISK OF PREDICTING FUTURE CARIES IN THE PERMANENT DENTITION

The potential benefit of identifying these 3 distinct patterns of dental caries in the pri-mary dentition is the ability to predict the risk of future dental caries. Caries risk assessment should be performed at a child's first dental visit and on a regular basis thereafter.[14] It is known from research following 362 Chinese children ages 3 years to 5 years for 8 years that children having dental caries in their primary teeth were 3 times more likely to develop caries in their permanent teeth.[23] The highest predictive value (85.4%) came from having caries on any of the primary molars. The highest sensitivity (93.9%) for prediction of dental caries in the permanent dentition was also from the presence of dental caries on any of the primary molars. Therefore, it be-hooves clinicians to aggressively institute prevention strategies after diagnosing ECC or LCC to protect the permanent dentition from experiencing dental caries.

LCC begins most often on the distal surface of the first primary molar and then in-volves the mesial surface of the second primary molar. Dean and colleagues[24] showed an association of 69% of primary molar teeth with proximal caries and caries on the adjacent proximal surface. They also reported that 89% of subjects who developed a proximal lesion on a primary molar in 1 quadrant developed another proximal lesion on a primary molar in another quadrant. Vanderas and colleagues[25] reported a posi-tive association between caries on the distal aspect of the second primary molar and mesial aspect of the corresponding first permanent molar, indicating progression of the disease to the permanent dentition. Once this disease is present in the permanent dentition, due to its chronic multifocal nature, multiple studies indicate there is a life-long interproximal caries risk.[23–25] Consequently, specific prevention strategies must be instituted to prevent caries lesion development in the interproximal area of primary teeth as well as to prevent repeating the pattern of interproximal lesions involving the permanent dentition.

It is well recognized that the development of MIH in the permanent first molars and permanent central incisors share similar mineralization timing.[26] Although the exact etiology of the hypomineralization is still unknown, repeated illnesses in the first years after birth show a strong correlation with occurrence of MIH. It is reasonable to assume if the illness is prolonged, then the mineralization of the second primary molars and the permanent first molars and incisors might be affected given the close proximity of their mineralization periods.[27,28] Therefore, PSMH with or without caries involvement may be an early warning sign of MIH in the permanent dentition. If PSMH is diagnosed, then it is important to be vigilant in monitoring the status of mineralization of the permanent incisors and first molars as soon after eruption for timely management and preservation of the permanent tooth structure.

SUMMARY

Accurate diagnosis of disease is the cornerstone to targeting precision-oriented prevention strategies as well as appropriately managing the disease state. This article describes 3 common patterns of dental caries in the primary dentition with distinct presentations: ECC, LCC, and PSMH-C. Each pattern has unique characteristics influencing both the therapeutic and preventive strategies. The overall goal is to protect the developing psyche of the child, stabilize or restore the dentition to health and natural esthetics when possible, and maintain space for the eruption of the permanent dentition while also respecting caregiver desires.

REFERENCES

1. Dye BA, Tan S, Smith V, et al. Trends in oral health status: United States. 1988-1994 and 1999-2004. Vital Health Stat 11 2007;248:1–92.
2. Duperon DF. Early childhood caries: a continuing dilemma. J Calif Dent Assoc 1995;23(2):15–22.
3. Berkowitz RJ. Causes, treatment and prevention of early childhood caries: a microbiologic perspective. J Can Dent Assoc 2003;69(5):304–7.
4. American Academy of Pediatric Dentistry. Policy on early childhood caries (ECC): classifications, consequences, and preventive strategies. Pediatr Dent 2018–2019; 40(6):60–2.
5. American Academy of Pediatric Dentistry. Policy on early childhood caries (ECC): unique challenges and treatment options. Pediatr Dent 2018–2019;40(6):63–4.
6. Ismail AI. Prevention of early childhood caries. Community Dent Oral Epidemiol 1998;26(Supplement 1):49–61.
7. Keels MA, Carney C, et al. Beyond ECC-Pediatric Dental Treatment Patterns. Poster session #1849 presented at IADR/AADR. Vancouver, June 21, 2019.
8. Hale KJ. American Academy of Pediatrics Section on Pediatric Dentistry. Oral health risk assessment timing and establishment of the dental home. Pediatrics 2003;111(5):1113–6.
9. American Academy of Pediatrics, Bright Futures Steering Committee. Promoting oral health. In: Hagan JF, Shaw JS, Duncan PM, editors. Bright futures: guidelines for health supervision of infants, children, and adolescents. 3rd edition. Elk Grove Village (IL): American Academy of Pediatrics; 2016. p. 205–16.
10. Twetman S. Caries prevention with fluoride toothpaste in children: an update. Eur Arch Paediatr Dent 2009;10(3):162–7.

11. American Dental Association Council on Scientific Affairs. Fluoride toothpaste use for young children. JADA 2014;145(2):1190–1.
12. Wright JT, Hanson N, Ristic H, et al. Fluoride toothpaste efficacy and safety in children younger than 6 years. J Am Dent Assoc 2014;145(2):182–9.
13. Hujoel PP, Cunha-Cruz J, Banting DW. Dental flossing and interproximal caries: a systematic review. J Dent Res 2006;85(4):298–305.
14. American Academy of Pediatric Dentistry. Caries-risk assessment and management for infants, children and adolescents. Pediatr Dent 2018–2019; 40(6):205–12.
15. U.S. Food and Drug Administration. Drug Safety Communication. FDA review results in new warnings about using general anesthetics and sedation drugs in young children and pregnant women. Available at: https://www.fda.gov/media/101937/download.
16. Slayton R, Urquhart O, Araujo MB, et al. Evidence-based clinical practice guideline on nonrestorative treatments for caries lesions: a report from the American Dental Association. J Am Dent Assoc 2018;149(10):837–49.
17. Kuhnisch J, Estrand KR, Pretty I, et al. Best clinical practice guideline for management of early caries lesions in children and young adults: an EAPD policy document. Eur Arch Paediatr Dent 2016;17(1):3–12.
18. American Academy of Pediatric Dentistry. Pediatric restorative dentistry. Pediatr Dent 2018-2019;40(6);330–42.
19. American Academy of Pediatric Dentistry. Management of the developing dentition and occulsion in pediatric dentistry. Pediatr Dent 2018–2019;40(6):352–65.
20. Fontana M, Gooch BF, Junger ML. The Hall technique may be an effective treatment modality for caries in primary molars. J Evid Based Dent Pract 2012;12(2): 110–2.
21. Santamaría RM, Innes NPT, Machiulskiene V, et al. Alternative caries management options for primary molars: 2.5-year outcomes of a randomised clinical trial. Caries Res 2018;51(6):605–14.
22. Coll JA, Seale NC, Vargas K, et al. Primary tooth vital pulp therapy: a systematic review and meta-analysis. Pediatr Dent 2017;39(1):16–27.
23. Li Y, Wang W. Predicting caries in permanent teeth from caries in primary teeth: an eight-year cohort study. J Dent Res 2002;81(8):561–6.
24. Dean JA, Barton DH, Vahedi I, et al. Progression of interproximal caries in the primary dentition. J Clin Pediatr Dent 1997;22(1):59–62.
25. Vanderas AP, Kavvadia K, Papagiannoulis L. Development of caries in permanent first molars adjacent to primary second molars with interproximal caries: four-year prospective radiographic study. Pediatr Dent 2004;26(4):362–8.
26. Schour I, Massler M. The development of the human dentition. J Am Dent Assoc 1941;20:379–427.
27. Weerheum KL. Molar incisor hypomineralisation (MIH). Eur Arch Paediatr Dent 2003;(3):1–6.
28. William V, Messer LB, Burrow MF. Molar incisor hypominerlization: review and recommendations for clinical management. Pediatr Dent 2006;28:224–32.

Personalized Dental Caries Management for Frail Older Adults and Persons with Special Needs

Leonardo Marchini, DDS, MSD, PhD[a],*,
Ronald Ettinger, BDS, MDS, DDSc, DDSc(hc)[b], Jennifer Hartshorn, DDS[c]

KEYWORDS

- Aged • Frail elderly • Developmental disabilities • Mental health • Dental caries
- Root caries • Oral health • Oral hygiene

KEY POINTS

- Frail older adults and persons with special needs include a diverse group of people with one or more disabilities that make them susceptible to rapid oral health deterioration (ROHD).
- The ROHD assessment helps practitioners determine the risk of oral health deterioration and identify how to deliver a personalized approach to dental care.
- ROHD risk factors are classified into three main categories: general health, social support, and oral conditions.
- ROHD risk levels are classified into four levels.

INTRODUCTION

The world's population is aging, and this trend is not only pronounced but also historically unprecedented.[1,2] In the next four decades, the world's older adults (customarily, older adults are persons older than age 65[a]) will increase from 800 million to 2

Disclosure Statement: The authors have nothing to disclose.
[a] Department of Preventive and Community Dentistry, The University of Iowa College of Dentistry and Dental Clinics, N337-1 Dental Science, Iowa City, IA 52242, USA; [b] Department of Prosthodontics, The University of Iowa College of Dentistry and Dental Clinics, N-409 Dental Science, Iowa City, IA 52242, USA; [c] Department of Preventive and Community Dentistry, The University of Iowa College of Dentistry and Dental Clinics, W327 Dental Science, Iowa City, IA 52242, USA
* Corresponding author.
E-mail address: leonardo-marchini@uiowa.edu

[a] However, aging has been defined as a biologic process and therefore older adults could be any person 21 years or older who may be biologically old.

https://doi.org/10.1016/j.cden.2019.06.003
0011-8532/19/© 2019 Elsevier Inc. All rights reserved.
dental.theclinics.com

billion people.[3] In general, the current cohort of older adults has been reported as healthier than previous ones. However, this progress has been unequal,[1,3] and older adults still have more extensive health problems that require more intense health care for longer periods of time than younger people. As a consequence, the number of people living with disabilities increases with age.[4] This poses an important challenge to health care systems around the globe.[1,3]

In conjunction with population aging, there is also an increasing number of younger adults living with disabilities, which occurred because of a reduced mortality rate among disabled children and adolescents. In the United States, 10.5% of people aged 18 to 64 had some type of disability in the year 2015.[4] The overall prevalence of people living with disabilities in the United States in 2015 was 12.6%, ranging from 9.9% in Utah to 19.4% in West Virginia.[4]

Oral diseases are still highly prevalent in the global and US aging population.[5] Because of population growth and aging, the cumulative burden of oral diseases has increased. Untreated caries in permanent teeth was the most prevalent chronic condition reported in 2015, affecting 2.5 billion people worldwide.[5] In industrialized countries, oral health has improved for older adults in the last few decades, resulting in lower prevalence rates of caries, periodontal disease, and edentulism when compared with previous cohorts.[6,7] However, the oral disease burden among older adults is still high,[6] and caries has been shown to be an active disease among this population[8] and even more so among frail older adults.[8,9] It is explained in part by the fact that more older adults retain their teeth into old age, and gingival recession exposes more tooth surfaces to the risk of root caries.[6,8,10] Thus, caries management among older adults should target preventing and controlling coronal and root caries, which has proved to be challenging.[10]

Adults living with disabilities are exposed to different risk factors that negatively impact their oral hygiene routines, and their ability to access dental care, and consequently increases their risk of caries. These risk factors include but are not limited to cognitive impairment,[11] dependence on caregivers,[12] polypharmacy,[13] poor manual dexterity,[14] financial constraints,[7] and xerostomia.[13,15] The influence of these risk factors makes controlling dental caries among this population even more challenging.

It is important to prevent the development of caries among frail older adults and persons with special needs to avoid infection, pain, and tooth loss. These consequences of caries have been shown to impact systemic health and quality of life.[16–19] To be successful in assessing and managing caries risk among these populations, one should consider all the patient modifying factors in a systematic way. In this article, the authors discuss how to provide a program of personalized and effective dental caries management for frail older adults and persons with special needs.

RAPID ORAL HEALTH DETERIORATION

Frail older adults and persons with special needs are composed of a wide diversity of people with different health problems, which require different types and intensities of care. In an initial attempt to help clinicians to determine the level of care necessary for different older adults, the aging population was classified into three groups: (1) functionally independent older adults, who can access oral health care on their own (70% of people older than age 65)[20]; (2) frail older adults, who can access oral health care with help from others (20% of people older than age 65)[20]; and (3) functionally dependent older adults, who benefit most if oral health care is provided in their place of residency (5% are homebound and 5% are nursing home residents).[20] This classification[b] proved to be important because each category requires a different philosophic approach to care, depending on the patient's modifying factors, which may range from the most sophisticated and technical treatment available to no treatment at all. More recently, Chi and Ettinger[21] presented a more extensive approach encompassing six distinct life periods, from early childhood to older adulthood, when discussing oral health–related issues with regard to caries prevention for people with special needs. A unifying approach that considers all risk factors for the entire population of frail older adults and persons with special needs is still lacking.

Recently, a systematic approach to teach dental students how to assess the risk of rapid oral health deterioration (ROHD) was introduced.[22] This approach used education theory to develop a learning guide aimed at reproducing the expert's thought process when assessing frail older adults or persons with special needs, and is also used by more experienced dental practitioners. The strategy depends on evidence-based risk factors collected from the dental literature that have been shown to increase the risk of ROHD. It also includes a learning guide to help the practitioner to evaluate the risk, present customized treatment alternatives, and communicate plans to patients and/or their caregivers.[22] The most common evidence-based ROHD risk factors among frail older adults and persons with special needs are described next.

RAPID ORAL HEALTH DETERIORATION RISK FACTORS

Evidence-based risk factors for ROHD is classified into three categories: (1) general health, (2) social support, and (3) oral conditions. These risk factors are also referred to as modifying factors (**Box 1**), and influence treatment decisions either independently or are multifactorial.

General Health

The ROHD risk factors in this category are usually collected by oral health providers through health history forms, medication lists, and the initial interview with the patient. For example, there are multiple diseases that reduce patients' ability to maintain a proper oral hygiene routine, and thus increase patients' likelihood of experiencing ROHD, such as congenital (ie, cerebral palsy) and acquired physical (ie, rheumatoid arthritis) deficits.

Patients' ability to keep adequate oral hygiene routines are limited by cognitive deficits,[23,24] because patients may not be able to remember to perform oral hygiene, do not know how to do it, or are not able to appreciate the importance of having good oral hygiene. Developmental disabilities, such as Down syndrome[25] and autism spectrum disorders,[26] can cause cognitive deficits. Later in life, such diseases as Alzheimer disease and other dementias[27] can also cause cognitive deficits. Additionally, cognitive deficits can prevent patients from communicating oral pain or discomfort, providing informed consent, adapting to dentures, and adhering to treatment and maintenance plans.[28]

Keeping good oral hygiene routines can also be more difficult for patients with functional deficits,[14] such as patients who have had a cerebrovascular accident,[14] patients who are quadriplegic,[29] have cerebral palsy,[29] and advanced Parkinson disease,[30] and also patients with severe osteoarthritis or rheumatoid arthritis.[14] Although some of these conditions may also have a cognitive component, manual dexterity is compromised even if there is no cognitive deficit, reducing the patients' capacity to perform appropriate oral hygiene by themselves (**Figs. 1** and **2**).

---

[b] This classification is based on national US disability data, but is similar in many industrialized Western countries.[4]

> **Box 1**
> **Rapid oral health deterioration risk factors**
>
> Risk Factors/Modifying factors
> 1. General health conditions
>   - Cognitive deficits: Alzheimer disease and other dementias
>   - Functional deficits: stroke, osteoarthritis, Parkinson disease, and so forth
>   - Sensory losses: speech, sight, hearing, and taste
>   - Medications: oral and systemic side effects, drug interactions
>   - Manageable chronic diseases: hypertension, diabetes, osteoporosis, and so forth
>   - Degree of dependence/autonomy: institutionalization, home care, dependence on caregivers, and so forth
>   - Terminal diseases/palliative care
>   - Life expectancy
> 2. Social support
>   - Institutional support
>   - Family/social support
>   - Financial issues: private insurance, Medicare, Medicaid, social security, and so forth
>   - Transportation
>   - Access to care
>   - Education and oral health literacy
>   - Informed consent
>   - Expectations
> 3. Oral conditions
>   - Oral hygiene: independency or dependency
>   - Periodontal condition
>   - Caries
>   - Number of teeth/restorations, number of chewing pairs
>   - Prosthetic status: fixed, removable, implants
>   - Oral lesions: inflammation, oral cancer
>   - Stop seeing the dentist

Some conditions/diseases predispose patients to more aggressive oral disease. Immunocompromising conditions,[31] such as AIDS, patient taking immune-suppressant drugs, or anticancer chemotherapeutic agents, and uncontrolled diabetes[32] are examples of conditions that predispose patients to more aggressive oral disease, thus increasing patients' risk of ROHD. Polypharmacy used to control different diseases and/or its symptoms can also lead to reduced salivary flow, which

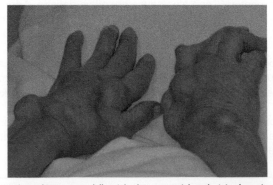

Fig. 1. Hands of a patient (67 years old) with rheumatoid arthritis showing the effects of the disease, which limits her manual dexterity.

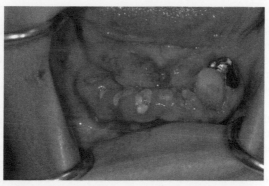

Fig. 2. ROHD caused by patient's inability to brush her teeth because of her rheumatoid arthritis.

is another condition that has been frequently linked to more aggressive oral disease among frail older adults and persons with special needs.[13,33,34]

Sensory impairments (mainly sight, hearing, taste, and proprioception) can also reduce patients' ability to perform appropriate oral hygiene. If patients cannot see, plaque removal may be incomplete, or if patients do not hear well they may not adhere to treatment maintenance plans because they do not fully understand what has been discussed. Taste and proprioceptive changes can impact patients' ability to adapt to dentures. Patients with autism spectrum disorders often present with sensory challenges that can benefit from appropriate sensory adaptations when providing dental care.[35]

Mental health conditions have also been shown to impair patients' capacity of maintaining appropriate oral hygiene, providing informed consent, and adhering to treatment and maintenance plans. Some of the important factors that might impact oral health care for patients with serious mental health conditions are the type and severity of the illness; mood, motivation, and self-esteem; lack of oral health perception; lack of self-discipline to maintain daily oral hygiene; and side effect of medications.[36] Destructive habits, such as smoking, poor diet, and substance abuse, are also common issues associated with people with mental disabilities.[37] Although poor oral health findings are common among people with mental health problems and many barriers for appropriate oral health care have been identified, no current investigation has identified enablers to improve oral health care.[37]

Among the different mental health diseases, depression is of special interest because it is particularly prevalent among older adults and can increase the risk for ROHD not only by discontinuing daily oral hygiene, but also because of the strong xerostomic effect of the use of antidepressants.[38] Another group of mental health conditions associated with increased risk of ROHD are the eating disorders, which can cause dental erosion. Dental erosion is also often seen associated with gastroesophageal reflux disease, which is prevalent among individuals with developmental disabilities.[39]

Providers should be aware that multiple general health-related risk factors are often found in frail older adults and patients with special needs, for instance survivors of a cerebrovascular accident may have concomitant cognitive and functional deficits. Also, depression is common in early dementia and these cognitive impairments may be by aggravated polypharmacy-induced xerostomia.

Social Support

Social support–related risk factors for ROHD are most commonly overlooked by oral health practitioners. Nevertheless, ROHD risk factors related to the patients' social support may play an important role in facilitating or making it more difficult for patients to access appropriate oral health care, maintain daily oral hygiene, and adhere to a proposed treatment plan.

Lack of income has been reported as an important barrier for health care use.[7,37] The families of frail older adults and patients with special needs have a higher economic burden as compared with families without members with special care needs,[7] therefore discretionary finances may not be available to access health care. In addition to treatment cost, paying for transportation and parking is an added barrier. In addition, lack of dental insurance has also been cited as another important barrier to care.[7,40]

Another social support–related risk factor is patients' dependency on caregivers, which is considered the major barrier for receiving appropriate daily oral hygiene and accessing oral health care.[12] Caregivers are anyone from a family member to a nursing aid, who provides care at the patient's home or in a long-term care facility. The level of care provided varies depending on the severity of the disability and the willingness of the patient to cooperate. Many factors have been reported to influence the provision of this care, including the caregivers' level of training[41] and their oral health literacy.[42,43] Institutionalization is another important risk factor for ROHD, because most of the long-term care facilities lack appropriate oral hygiene routines[9,44] and have been resistant to many different strategies suggested to improve the provision of oral care.[9,45]

Community-level factors that should be considered as risk factors of ROHD include access to community water fluoridation, healthy foods (including buying, preparing, and eating), and access to dental providers with appropriate training.[21]

Other important risk factors related to social support are the stigma and prejudice against frail older adults and persons with special needs. Stigma related to people with mental conditions has been reported as a significant barrier for accessing adequate care.[37] Ageism (defined as "the stereotyping, prejudice and discrimination toward people based on age")[46] has also been described by the World Health Organization as one of the most important barriers for providing age-appropriate care for the growing number of older adults.[47] Ageism has been shown to be pervasive among health professions,[48] and dentistry is no exception.[49,50]

The lack of interprofessional collaborative practice among health care providers has been cited[37] as a barrier for receiving appropriate care for frail older adults and persons with special needs. For these patients, it is important to assess how they function in their environment and how dentistry fits into their lifestyle and overall treatment/management goals. To make these assessments requires interprofessional collaboration, which is necessary to integrate several different disciplines to achieve good outcomes. Because these patients often have a multitude of health conditions, each requiring unique therapies and different providers, communication between providers is necessary to understand the patient's needs and prevent overtreatment or undertreatment.

Oral Conditions

Some oral health conditions encountered among frail older adults and persons with special needs can also increase their risk for ROHD. Xerostomia is a common oral health condition that predisposes patients to oral health decline, and is usually caused by polypharmacy.[13,33,34,51] Other causes for xerostomia include systemic diseases (eg, diabetes), psychoaffective disorders, head and neck radiation, and autoimmune diseases (eg, Sjögren syndrome).[51]

It is important to realize the difference between xerostomia, which is the subjective symptom of having a dry mouth reported by the patient, and salivary gland hypofunction, which is the reduced salivary flow that is measured by quantifying the amount of saliva produced in a given time.[34] It is advisable to measure xerostomia and salivary gland hypofunction in a patient where xerostomia is contributing to ROHD. Thus, a question about dry mouth sensation in the patient health history can help determine the need for assessing salivary flow output.[34]

Xerostomia prevalence among older adults ranges from 12% to 39%, with a weighted average of 21%, which shows xerostomia is a common condition in this population. The prevalence of xerostomia among younger adults is estimated to be about half of that compared with older adults. Xerostomia impacts patient speech, taste, swallowing, eating, and wearing dentures. Additionally, xerostomia can also contribute to halitosis, burning mouth sensation, and increases the caries risk.[34]

In addition to xerostomia, other oral conditions can also lead to an increased caries risk. Among older adults, the cumulative nature of gingival recession and consequent root surface exposure in later life is a major risk factor for root surface caries. Other risk factors include poor plaque control and previous experience with coronal and root caries.[15,52] Wearing partial dentures[53] and having a heavily restored dentition[10] are also risk factors for ROHD. Among younger adults with special needs, enamel defects, which is associated with some developmental disabilities,[54] have also been linked to increased caries risk and further ROHD.[55] Another local risk factor is the use of liquid medications with high sugar content for patients who are unable to swallow tablets.[56]

RAPID ORAL HEALTH DETERIORATION RISK ASSESSMENT

The ROHD risk assessment was designed on the premise that patients with disabilities can have a combination of risk factors, which can lead to a rapid decline in oral health. Because of the complexity of their health conditions, older adults and patients with special needs who have a high caries prevalence may not improve their oral health by simply instructing the patients to brush their teeth. It is only with a complete understanding of all the risk factors affecting a patient that caries risk can be improved, treatment can be effectively provided, and prevention can be improved. The assessment of the ROHD risk and selection of appropriate course of treatment to deter or manage the risk can be done in a systematic way.[22]

The first step is gathering information concerning ROHD risk factors. At this point, the oral health provider should be able to assess the completeness of the data gathered from the patient/caregiver interview, health history form, medication list, intraoral examination and radiographic evidence, and from the caries risk assessment. If any important information regarding one of the three categories of risk factors (ie, general health, social support, and oral conditions) is missing, it should be supplemented at this time.

The second step prioritizes the already gathered information. From all the general health conditions, social support factors, and oral health conditions presented by the patient, the clinician needs to decide which ones are more likely to contribute to ROHD progression and help determine the treatment plan. For example, if an adult patient with Down syndrome presents with controlled type II diabetes mellitus and is able to carry out his/her own daily oral hygiene at a reasonable level, it is less likely that diabetes will influence oral disease progression and modify the treatment plan. But if the same patient presents with signs of early dementia, this information is likely to increase the patient's risk for ROHD and also influence the treatment plan to increase preventive measures and recruit future caregivers to help with oral hygiene, because self-care is expected to decline as the dementia progresses.

The third step categorizes the patient's current ROHD stage to predict the future oral health of the patient if no dental treatment is provided, or whether an alternative treatment approach may be needed. This step helps the provider to understand and manage the patient's disease as a continuum, and therefore there is a need to explain to the patient and the caregiver the importance of the dental treatment plan. As a guide for the oral health provider, ROHD is classified into four categories depending on the severity of the risk factors and the disease progression:

1. Risk factors are not present, therefore no ROHD is occurring
2. Risk factors are present, however, ROHD is not currently occurring
3. Risk factors are present, and ROHD is currently occurring
4. Risk factors are present, and ROHD has already occurred

This ROHD classification helps determine the preventive and restorative approaches needed in the treatment plan. However, there are often no clear demarcations between the stages, and patients may be transitioning from one stage to another. Therefore, thinking about risk factors as they relate to disease progression and how they impact treatment planning for a given patient is the emphasis of this step.

The fourth step identifies the treatment alternatives, recommending a specific intervention with a rationale, and then developing a communication plan for the patient, caregivers, and other members of the health care team. These topics are discussed in further detail in the next section of this article. **Box 2** summarizes treatment planning using the ROHD assessment.

RAPID ORAL HEALTH DETERIORATION MANAGEMENT STRATEGIES FOR CARIES PREVENTION AMONG FRAIL OLDER ADULTS AND PERSONS WITH SPECIAL NEEDS
Caries Prevention Strategies

Caries prevention is included in all four levels of ROHD. Caries prevention strategy should be in place for patients not experiencing ROHD, so they do not experience ROHD in their lifetime. For those experiencing ROHD, prevention should also be included to avoid further progression of ROHD. For patients for whom ROHD has

---

Box 2
Treatment planning using the ROHD assessment

Step 1. Gathering information concerning ROHD risk factors

Step 2. Prioritizing the information (What matters most?)

Step 3. Categorizes risk for ROHD
   ROHD risk categories
   1. Risk factors are not present, therefore no ROHD is occurring
   2. Risk factors are present, however, ROHD is not currently occurring
   3. Risk factors are present, and ROHD is currently occurring
   4. Risk factors are present, and ROHD has already occurred
   What will happen if I do nothing?

Step 4. Identify possible treatment alternatives

already happened but some teeth can still be used as abutments, caries prevention is crucial for maintaining these abutment teeth. For edentulous patients, caries prevention does not apply, but it is important to remember that oral hygiene is still needed to prevent local inflammation and infection. Therefore, the most important caries prevention strategies that relate to common risk factors in this population are described in the following paragraphs.

Impact of dry mouth and its management

Dry mouth can have a severe impact on caries risk, because the salivary protective system (including salivary buffers, antimicrobial activity, and calcium and phosphate replenishment) is reduced.[51] When treating patients presenting with dry mouth, the oral health provider should keep in mind the following aspects of dry mouth management: (1) hydration (dehydrated patients produce less saliva), (2) symptoms relief (relief of the discomfort caused by the lack of moisture and lubrication), (3) managing problems with dentures (saliva is important to retain and comfortably wear dentures), (4) monitoring the use of medication (medication reconciliation[c] may reduce the xerostomic effect of some drugs), and (5) preventing soft tissue damage and dental caries **(Figs. 3–5)**.[34]

A broader approach should include maintaining appropriate hydration, using saliva stimulants or saliva substitutes (liquids or gel), and revaluating the patient's medications to reduce the xerostomic effect of their prescribed medications. These steps can help reduce the patients' oral discomfort caused by dry mouth and improve the quality of their lives.

Dehydration is prevalent among frail older adults and persons with special needs but there is a lack of awareness about this condition among patients and caregivers.[57] Unfortunately, patients when educated to sip liquids throughout the day may opt to use sugar-rich beverages or soda, increasing their caries risk. Therefore, it is important to educate patients and caregivers about the importance of drinking water, which has multiple benefits, such as keeping an adequate fluid intake, reducing the dry mouth sensation, and avoiding increased caries risk.[57]

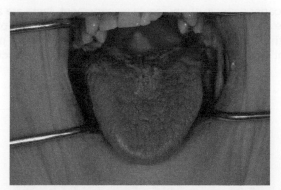

Fig. 3. Patient (69 years old) presenting with dry mouth because of polypharmacy.

---

[c] "Medication reconciliation is the process of creating the most accurate list possible of all medications a patient is taking—including drug name, dosage, frequency, and route—and comparing that list against the physician's admission, transfer, and/or discharge orders, with the goal of providing correct medications to the patient" (http://www.ihi.org/Topics/ADEsMedicationReconciliation/Pages/default.aspx).

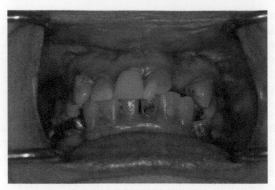

Fig. 4. Multiple carious lesions associated with dry mouth in the patient shown in **Fig. 3**.

For patients with residual secretory capacity, the use of saliva stimulants, such as chewing xylitol gums or using lozenges, and parasympathetic drugs can help improve salivary flow (eg, pilocarpine, bethanechol, and anethole trithione).[51] Saliva substitutes are usually presented as a gel, oral rinses, or sprays, and can help reduce dry mouth sensation and associated oral discomfort.[58] Oral discomfort can also be reduced by having a less spicy and less acidic diet, and using oral hygiene products, such as toothpastes and oral rinses specific for patients with dry mouth that have less flavoring agents (eg, peppermint and menthol) and are sodium lauryl sulfate–free.[59]

Frail older adults and persons with special needs are often taking multiple medications,[9,33] and most of the time xerostomia among this population is caused by polypharmacy.[51] Reconciling medication lists can help improve patients' health outcomes, reducing adverse drug reactions and reducing costs.[60] In an interprofessional collaborative practice where the dentist can present the effects of xerostomia on patients' quality of life, the xerostomic effects of drugs can also be considered when reconciling a patient medication list, potentially helping to reduce dry mouth.

Besides the broader aspects of dry mouth management, there are also some other strategies that are specifically designed to reduce caries risk among patients presenting with dry mouth. These strategies should be customized for each patient, depending on the patient's risk factors, and their ability to follow the prescribed therapies.

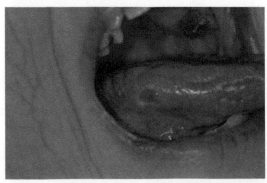

Fig. 5. Traumatic ulceration of the right border of the tongue related to lack of lubrication caused by dry mouth in the patient shown in **Fig. 3**.

Some of the tools that are deployed to help reduce caries risk for patients with xerostomia include remineralizing products, fluoride, and antibacterial products.

A remineralizing product often found beneficial for patients with xerostomia is Recaldent (casein-phosphopeptide–stabilized amorphous calcium phosphate nanocomplexes), which is the active ingredient of the MI Paste (GC America, Alsip, IL). MI Paste supplies calcium and phosphate to saliva, thus helping remineralization. It is easily applied to the tooth surface using fingertips after brushing. When applied at night, it also provides some moisturizing capacity because of casein. Although MI Paste does not contain fluoride, it has been added to MI Paste Plus (GC America).[61]

Fluoride exposure occurs from many sources, such as fluoridated water; self-applied sources, such as over-the-counter toothpastes, prescription/high-concentration (5000 ppm) toothpastes, and fluoridated rinses; and professionally applied sources, such as silver diamine fluoride (SDF), fluoride varnishes, and fluoride gel.[62] Patients with xerostomia can benefit from a higher fluoride exposure to reduce their caries risk. However, many toothpastes contain a detergent, sodium lauryl sulfate. This detergent can cause a burning sensation for those patients who have xerostomia. Therefore, over-the-counter fluoride toothpastes and prescription toothpastes without sodium lauryl sulfate should be recommended. A recommended approach that has been used in patients with xerostomia is a combination of prescribing 5000 ppm toothpaste to be used twice a day and have the patient returning for regular recalls every 3 months for fluoride varnish application.[51] It is critical to instruct patients and caregivers not to rinse after brushing with 5000 ppm toothpaste, but simply to spit. (See Margherita Fontana's article, "Nonrestorative Management of Cavitated and Noncavitated Caries Lesions," in this issue.)

Oral physiotherapy (aids for tooth brushing and flossing)
Daily mechanical removal of plaque is important for controlling bacterial load and reducing dental plaque. People who brush their teeth infrequently have higher incidence and increments of carious lesions.[63] However, many frail older adults and persons with special needs are not able to independently brush their teeth. Some patients are not able to brush because of cognitive deficits, and these patients need to be reminded to brush, or to be supervised while brushing; and some need a caregiver to brush for them. Another group of patients may be cognitively intact, but do not have the manual dexterity to brush by themselves. Depending on the severity of the patient disability, some patients in this group may benefit from larger toothbrush handles and/or electric toothbrushes, whereas other patients need help from a caregiver.

A larger toothbrush handle can allow patients with impaired manual dexterity to brush their own teeth, and several techniques have been described to fabricate customized toothbrush handles.[64] Toothbrush handles can also be improvised from bicycle handles, perforated rubber balls or a piece of swimming noodle. Power toothbrushes have larger handles in addition of being more effective for plaque removal,[65] particularly for frail older adults and persons with special needs.[66,67]

For caregivers who provide daily oral hygiene, the most appropriate tool will vary depending on patients' systemic conditions, cooperation and preferences. Regular toothbrushes with bent heads may help to hold the cheeks and lips apart, and provide better access. Some patients will benefit from caregivers using mouth props to help keep the patients' mouths open. Many patients can benefit from having a caretaker use a power toothbrush, although some patients with cognitive deficits are afraid/annoyed because of the vibration and/or the sounds.

Fluoride

(See Margherita Fontana's article, "Nonrestorative Management of Cavitated and Noncavitated Caries Lesions," in this issue.)

For patients with higher risk of developing caries, increasing their exposure to fluoride can help arrest caries progression and prevent new lesions. For these adult patients, a regimen of using 5000 ppm fluoride toothpaste twice a day and applying fluoride varnish every 3 to 6 months has been recommended.[68] Another protocol is daily use of 0.09% fluoride rinse followed by professional application of 1.23% fluoride gel every 3 to 6 months. However, the rinses are not as easy to use among frail older adults and persons with special needs because the rinse can be swallowed by patients with cognitive deficits and it is difficult for patients with physical deficits to swish and spit a rinse. Furthermore, the gel needs to stay into patients' mouth for 4 minutes, which is difficult for this population.

Another topical fluoride product is SDF, which has been used for a long time in many countries to arrest and prevent caries. This product has been available in the US market since 2014. The proportions of active ingredients in the SDF aqueous solution in the United States are 24% to 27% silver, 7.5% to 11.0% ammonia, and 5% to 6% fluoride.[69] Silver ions have an antibacterial effect, causing destruction of the cell wall, denaturizing cytoplasmic enzymes, and inhibiting DNA replication. Fluoride and ammonia have been linked to improved remineralization and formation of fluorapatite.[70]

For SDF application, targeted teeth should be isolated with cotton-rolls, dried with a triple syringe (or cotton pellet), then SDF is applied to the desired area using a microbrush for about a minute if possible, and the excess should be removed using cotton pellet.[71] Therefore, SDF application is technically easy, inexpensive, and has been proved to be safe[71] and effective for caries prevention and arresting caries among frail older adults[72,73] and persons with special needs.[74] One of the contraindications to use SDF is silver allergy, and the most negative side effect is darkening of the carious lesion, which may be important for some patients, mainly when involving anterior teeth.

Dietary changes for preventing caries

Meeting the diet and nutritional needs of frail older adults and persons with special needs is crucial for the maintenance of health, functional independence and quality of life. Persons with poor general health may experience difficulties in meeting their nutritional needs.[75] The existence of dental caries is strongly related to the consumption of sugar, and so by controlling the amount of sugar intake one can help reduce caries rates.[76] Also, oral health problems have been related to an inadequate diet among older adults,[77] and by improving diet quality it has been shown that root caries risk is reduced among older adults.[78] For instance, increasing vegetables and total grains intake has been shown to reduce root caries increments, whereas increasing consumption of sugar-sweetened carbonated beverages increases root caries increments.[78] Therefore, diet is an important factor to control caries risk among frail older adults and persons with special needs. Oral health care providers should educate patients and caregivers about the importance of having an adequate diet and reducing sugar consumption. However, just providing knowledge may not be sufficient to achieve behavior changes, because frail older adults and persons with special needs may lack the ability to apply the acquired knowledge to change their habits. In these circumstances, working with other members of the health care team may be necessary to induce behavior change. (See Teresa A. Marshall's article, "Dietary Implications for Dental Caries: a Practical Approach on Dietary Counseling," in this issue.)

Other preventive approaches
Replacing sugar with xylitol reduces caries risk by decreasing the amount of acid produced by acidogenic bacteria[51]; however, there is no strong evidence that xylitol-containing products can prevent caries.[79] Chlorhexidine in different formats has not been shown to be effective in caries prevention,[80,81] thus its use as the only method for caries control is not warranted.[51]

CARIES RESTORATIVE TREATMENT

(See Leo Tjäderhane and Arzu Tezvergil-Mutluay's article, "Performance of Adhesives and Restorative Materials After Selective Removal of Carious Lesions: Restorative Materials with Anticaries Properties," in this issue.)

Incomplete Caries Removal

International consensus has accepted the concepts of minimally invasive dental procedures, and it is considered the best practice to manage and control caries and to preserve hard tissues and keep the natural dentition.[82] This means that restoring a caries lesion should be done when it is not possible or desirable to arrest the existing lesion, and the focus should be on using all the preventive methods cited to control the disease and avoid further progression of existing lesions and/or the emergence of new lesions.

When a restorative approach is inevitable, the dentist's priorities should be to preserve healthy tooth structure, to remineralize natural tooth structure, and to obtain clear margins for a good restorative seal. This philosophy should stress the pulp as little as possible, and maximize the success of the restoration, and the survival of the tooth. Within this concept, infected or demineralized tissue does not need to be completely removed, whereas carious tissues are removed only to the extent needed to allow for a good seal of the restoration. In shallower lesions, distant from the pulp, selective removal to firm dentine should be carried out; whereas in deeper lesions, close to the pulp, selective removal to soft dentine has been shown to be successful.[82]

A range of different materials is used to restore teeth. Amalgam has been successfully used for a long period of time with some antibacterial properties against cariogenic bacteria.[82] However, resistance has emerged because of esthetic and environmental issues, and the use of composite resins has increased. Although composites in general have a similar longevity to amalgam,[83] composites are more susceptible to secondary caries in high-risk patients.[82]

When using composites, the dentist should keep in mind that bond strength is proportional to the area of the bonded surface to sound hard tissues, and therefore carious tissue that was left to protect the pulp from exposure should not be located at the margins of the preparation, which need to be on healthy tissue to allow for appropriate sealing.[82]

Glass ionomer cements (GIC) have been used as a third alternative for direct restorations. GICs were initially considered as a temporary material, but the most recent high-viscosity GICs have resulted in better longevity, comparable with composites or amalgams.[82] Glass ionomers are more biocompatible, release fluoride, adhere to dentine and enamel, and are becoming less technique sensitive. They are now commonly used as liners for deep restorations, and where moisture control is a problem. Resin-modified GIC has proved to be superior for use in cervical lesions.[84] GIC can also be used in combination with composite for open and closed sandwich techniques.[85] Because of its versatility, GICs are often used for frail older adults and persons with special needs, where the conditions for placing restorations are technically difficult. For example, GICs are a good alternative for restoring root caries, which often spreads below the gingival margin (**Figs. 6** and **7**).[85]

In a recent assessment of the longevity of 9184 dental restorations after 15 years, placed in a clinic dedicated to caring for frail older adults and persons with special needs, the following was found. Failing restorations numbered 28.7%, and the overall restoration life span was 6.2 years. Multivariable regression models showed that the greater the number of restorative surfaces the shorter the life span, and that restorations placed earlier in a patient's life lasted longer than subsequent restorations.[86]

Atraumatic Restorative Treatment

Atraumatic restorative treatment (ART) usually consists of manual soft caries excavation followed by high-viscosity GIC restorations under cotton-roll isolation. Because of its simplicity, ART reduces patient anxiety and discomfort during dental treatment. Therefore, ART has been successfully used among frail older adults and persons with special needs, and survival rates of teeth restored by ART are similar to conventional restorative techniques.[87] ART is particularly useful when providing care outside the dental office for frail older adults and persons with special needs or to patients with limited cooperation in the dental chair. It also has been shown to be cost-effective[88] and well-accepted by patients.[89]

Behavior Management

Many frail older adults and persons with special needs, especially those with mental health issues and/or cognitive deficits, can have a difficult time sitting in a dental chair, or having their teeth cleaned at home. Combative and aggressive patients can pose a risk to themselves, their caregivers, and their health care providers. Multiple types of challenging behavior can happen, such as refusing oral care, inability to understand what is happening, inability to follow directions, and physical aggressions (kicks, hits, bites).

Basic communication techniques should always be used by the provider, and they include being patient, respectful, and gentle; using patient's name; smiling, keeping eye contact, and moving slowly; introducing yourself; using plain language and short sentences; explaining what is going to be done and why; repeating instructions if

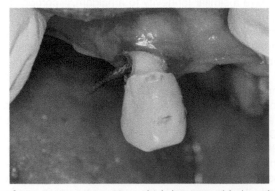

Fig. 6. Preparation for restoring root caries, which has spread below the gingival margin, resulting in difficulties with moisture control. A cord was placed to allow access for subgingival restoration.

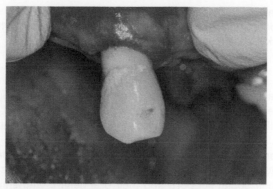

Fig. 7. Final restoration of the root caries shown in **Fig. 6**, with a high-viscosity glass ionomer.

necessary with neutral tone; and breaking down the instructions into single commands. It is important to always be polite, provide encouragement, and give positive feedback. If not successful, try a different time, because patients may react differently at different times of the day.[90]

More advanced techniques are presented in a mobile app (GeriaDental) that is downloaded for free, and can also be used by family and professional caregivers. The app is easily found in app stores for Apple and Android devices.

COMMUNICATION PLAN FOR THE PATIENT AND/OR CAREGIVER

Frail older adults and patients with special needs often present with a variety of comorbidities and functional impairments. Evaluating the needs of these patients requires thoughtful assessments from multidisciplinary health professionals. Therefore, providing the patient, caregivers, and occasionally other health care team members with a summary of the oral health findings, the proposed treatment plan with a rationale, and the strategies for the oral hygiene care required for maintaining patients oral health is of paramount importance for the long-term success of the therapy.[22]

The challenge of having multiple persons involved, who have different expectations and different perspectives, requires the oral health care provider to communicate effectively with all persons involved. The dentist needs to keep in mind how the perspectives of each individual may differ, and needs to determine who is responsible for the primary health care of the patient. The dentist needs to identify the various members of the health care team, understand their roles, and be part of the overall treatment goals. Therefore, information from all health care providers should be gathered during the initial interviews with patient and other members of the health care team. A multidisciplinary conference to assess the patient's needs would be ideal, but unfortunately rarely happens, except in certain institutions that are devoted to person-centered care.

Of particular importance is the communication with the patient's guardians/caretakers. If a patient is not able to provide informed consent, or even if he/she is capable but has an established guardian, the oral health care provider should also keep in mind that some patients may have a power-of-attorney for health and a different one for finances. Both parties must be consulted and their approval obtained before dental treatment. More about informed consent is found in the work by Kristen Flick and

Leonardo Marchini's article, "The Interprofessional Role in Dental Caries Management: From the Social Worker Perspective", in this issue, which is presented from a social worker's perspective.

SUMMARY

Frail older adults and people with special needs include a diverse group of people with different disabilities that make this group more susceptible to ROHD. Caries is a leading cause of ROHD. Therefore, it is important to consider the patient as a whole, and avoid a narrower, tooth-focused perspective.

To have a patient-centered perspective, it is necessary to consider each patient's personal characteristics. These include the patient's risk factors related to their general health, their social support, and their oral health. Gathering and analyzing these risk factors will help oral health providers to assess patients' risk for ROHD. Assessing the risk of ROHD helps determine how much preventive versus restorative treatment will be necessary, thereby helping providers think about the risk factors as they relate to disease progression and treatment planning. Some of the most important preventive caries management strategies for frail older adults and people with special needs include management of dry mouth problems, improvement of daily oral hygiene, use of different fluoride products, and dietary changes. Caries restorative treatment strategies commonly used among this group include incomplete caries removal, ART, and different techniques to help manage behavioral challenges.

Having a better understanding of the patient as a whole also can improve the oral health provider's ability to meaningfully communicate treatment and maintenance plans to the patient, his/her caregivers, and other members of the health care team. This is a necessary step, because patient adherence to appropriate maintenance is important for the long-term success of oral health treatment among frail older adults and people with special needs.

REFERENCES

1. WHO. World report on ageing and health. Geneva: World Health Organization; 2015. p. 260.

2. United_Nations, editor. World population prospects: the 2017 revision. New York: United Nations; 2017.

3. Bloom DE, Chatterji S, Kowal P, et al. Macroeconomic implications of population ageing and selected policy responses. Lancet 2015;385(9968):649–57.

4. Kraus L. 2016 disability statistics annual report. Durham (NH): University of New Hampshire; 2017.

5. Kassebaum NJ, Smith AGC, Bernabe E, et al. Global, regional, and national prevalence, incidence, and disability-adjusted life years for oral conditions for 195 countries, 1990-2015: a systematic analysis for the global burden of diseases, injuries, and risk factors. J Dent Res 2017;96(4):380–7.

6. Lopez R, Smith PC, Gostemeyer G, et al. Ageing, dental caries and periodontal diseases. J Clin Periodontol 2017;44(Suppl 18):S145–52.

7. Friedman PK, Kaufman LB, Karpas SL. Oral health disparity in older adults: dental decay and tooth loss. Dent Clin North Am 2014;58(4):757–70.

8. Thomson W. Epidemiology of oral health conditions in older people. Gerodontology 2014;31:9–16.

9. Marchini L, Recker E, Hartshorn J, et al. Iowa nursing facility oral hygiene (IN-FOH) intervention: a clinical and microbiological pilot randomized trial. Spec Care Dentist 2018;38(6):345–55.

10. Jablonski RY, Barber MW. Restorative dentistry for the older patient cohort. Br Dent J 2015;218(6):337–42.

11. Ni Chroinin D, Montalto A, Jahromi S, et al. Oral health status is associated with common medical comorbidities in older hospital inpatients. J Am Geriatr Soc 2016;64(8):1696–700.

12. Marchini L, Vieira PC, Bossan TP, et al. Self-reported oral hygiene habits among institutionalised elderly and their relationship to the condition of oral tissues in Taubaté, Brazil. Gerodontology 2006;23(1):33–7.

13. Singh ML, Papas A. Oral implications of polypharmacy in the elderly. Dent Clin North Am 2014;58(4):783–96.

14. Tavares M, Lindefjeld Calabi KA, San Martin L. Systemic diseases and oral health. Dent Clin North Am 2014;58(4):797–814.

15. Hayes M, Da Mata C, Cole M, et al. Risk indicators associated with root caries in independently living older adults. J Dent 2016;51:8–14.

16. Gil-Montoya JA, de Mello AL, Barrios R, et al. Oral health in the elderly patient and its impact on general well-being: a nonsystematic review. Clin Interv Aging 2015; 10:461–7.

17. Tan H, Peres KG, Peres MA. Retention of teeth and oral health-related quality of life. J Dent Res 2016;95(12):1350–7.

18. Ramsay SE, Whincup PH, Watt RG, et al. Burden of poor oral health in older age: findings from a population-based study of older British men. BMJ Open 2015; 5(12):e009476.

19. Tanaka T, Takahashi K, Hirano H, et al. Oral frailty as a risk factor for physical frailty and mortality in community-dwelling elderly. J Gerontol A Biol Sci Med Sci 2018;73(12):1661–7.

20. Ettinger RL, Beck JD. The new elderly: what can the dental profession expect? Spec Care Dentist 1982;2(2):62–9.

21. Chi DL, Ettinger RL. Prevention and nonsurgical management of dental caries over the life course for individuals with special health care needs. J Calif Dent Assoc 2014;42(7):455–63.

22. Marchini L, Hartshorn JE, Cowen H, et al. A teaching tool for establishing risk of oral health deterioration in elderly patients: development, implementation, and evaluation at a U.S. dental school. J Dent Educ 2017;81(11):1283–90.

23. Brennan LJ, Strauss J. Cognitive impairment in older adults and oral health considerations: treatment and management. Dent Clin North Am 2014;58(4): 815–28.

24. Chen X, Xie XJ, Yu L. The pathway from cognitive impairment to caries in older adults: a conceptual model. J Am Dent Assoc 2018;149(11):967–75.

25. Mubayrik AB. The dental needs and treatment of patients with Down syndrome. Dent Clin North Am 2016;60(3):613–26.

26. Chandrashekhar S, S Bommangoudar J. Management of autistic patients in dental office: a clinical update. Int J Clin Pediatr Dent 2018;11(3):219–27.

27. Delwel S, Binnekade TT, Perez RS, et al. Oral health and orofacial pain in older people with dementia: a systematic review with focus on dental hard tissues. Clin Oral Investig 2017;21(1):17–32.

28. Chen X, Zimmerman S, Potter GG, et al. Assessment of dentally related function in individuals with cognitive impairment: the dental activities test. J Am Geriatr Soc 2017;65(3):580–5.

29. de Carvalho RB, Mendes RF, Prado RR Jr, et al. Oral health and oral motor function in children with cerebral palsy. Spec Care Dentist 2011;31(2):58–62.

30. Barbe AG, Bock N, Derman SH, et al. Self-assessment of oral health, dental health care and oral health-related quality of life among Parkinson's disease patients. Gerodontology 2017;34(1):135–43.

31. Goldman KE. Dental management of patients with bone marrow and solid organ transplantation. Dent Clin North Am 2006;50(4):659–76, viii.

32. Eke PI, Thornton-Evans GO, Wei L, et al. Periodontitis in US adults: National Health and Nutrition Examination Survey 2009-2014. J Am Dent Assoc 2018; 149(7):576–88.e6.

33. Deco CPd, Reis MRVS, Marchini AMPdS, et al. Taste alteration, mouth dryness and teeth staining as side effects of medications taken by elderly. Braz J Oral Sci 2014;13(4):257–60.

34. Thomson WM. Dry mouth and older people. Aust Dent J 2015;60(Suppl 1):54–63.

35. Cermak SA, Stein Duker LI, Williams ME, et al. Sensory adapted dental environments to enhance oral care for children with autism spectrum disorders: a randomized controlled pilot study. J Autism Dev Disord 2015;45(9): 2876–88.

36. Clark DB. Mental health issues and special care patients. Dent Clin North Am 2016;60(3):551–66.

37. Slack-Smith L, Hearn L, Scrine C, et al. Barriers and enablers for oral health care for people affected by mental health disorders. Aust Dent J 2017;62(1):6–13.

38. Kisely S, Sawyer E, Siskind D, et al. The oral health of people with anxiety and depressive disorders: a systematic review and meta-analysis. J Affect Disord 2016;200:119–32.

39. Rada RE. Dental erosion due to GERD in patients with developmental disabilities: case theory. Spec Care Dentist 2014;34(1):7–11.

40. Edelstein BL. Engaging the U.S. Congress in the oral health of special-needs adults: lessons from pediatric oral health policy. Spec Care Dentist 2013;33(4): 198–203.

41. Barbosa CS, Marchini AM, Marchini L. General and oral health-related quality of life among caregivers of Parkinson's disease patients. Geriatr Gerontol Int 2013; 13(2):429–36.

42. Shah AH, Naseem M, Khan MS, et al. Oral health knowledge and attitude among caregivers of special needs patients at a comprehensive rehabilitation centre: an analytical study. Ann Stomatol (Roma) 2017;8(3):110–6.

43. de Lugt-Lustig KH, Vanobbergen JN, van der Putten GJ, et al. Effect of oral healthcare education on knowledge, attitude and skills of care home nurses: a systematic literature review. Community Dent Oral Epidemiol 2014;42(1): 88–96.

44. De Visschere LM, Grooten L, Theuniers G, et al. Oral hygiene of elderly people in long-term care institutions: a cross-sectional study. Gerodontology 2006;23(4): 195–204.

45. van der Putten GJ, Mulder J, de Baat C, et al. Effectiveness of supervised implementation of an oral health care guideline in care homes; a single-blinded cluster randomized controlled trial. Clin Oral Investig 2013;17(4):1143–53.

46. Officer A, de la Fuente-Nunez V. A global campaign to combat ageism. Bull World Health Organ 2018;96(4):295–6.

47. Prince MJ, Wu F, Guo Y, et al. The burden of disease in older people and implications for health policy and practice. Lancet 2015;385(9967):549–62.

48. Lloyd-Sherlock PG, Ebrahim S, McKee M, et al. Institutional ageism in global health policy. BMJ 2016;354:i4514.
49. Rucker R, Barlow PB, Hartshorn J, et al. Development and preliminary validation of an ageism scale for dental students. Spec Care Dentist 2018;38(1):31–5.
50. Rucker R, Barlow PB, Hartshorn J, et al. Dual institution validation of an ageism scale for dental students. Spec Care Dentist 2019;39(1):28–33.
51. Su N, Marek CL, Ching V, et al. Caries prevention for patients with dry mouth. J Can Dent Assoc 2011;77:b85.
52. Ritter AV, Preisser JS, Puranik CP, et al. A predictive model for root caries incidence. Caries Res 2016;50(3):271–8.
53. Mengatto CM, Marchini L, Bernardes LA, et al. Partial denture metal framework may harbor potentially pathogenic bacteria. J Adv Prosthodont 2015;7(6): 468–74.
54. Erika V, Modrić, Verzak Ž, et al. Developmental defects of enamel in children with intellectual disability. Acta Stomatol Croat 2016;50(1):65–71.
55. Vargas-Ferreira F, Salas MM, Nascimento GG, et al. Association between developmental defects of enamel and dental caries: a systematic review and meta-analysis. J Dent 2015;43(6):619–28.
56. Donaldson M, Goodchild JH, Epstein JB. Sugar content, cariogenicity, and dental concerns with commonly used medications. J Am Dent Assoc 2015;146(2): 129–33.
57. Abdallah L, Remington R, Houde S, et al. Dehydration reduction in community-dwelling older adults: perspectives of community health care providers. Res Gerontol Nurs 2009;2(1):49–57.
58. Jose A, Atassi M, Shneyer L, et al. A randomized clinical trial to measure mouth moisturization and dry mouth relief in dry mouth subjects using dry mouth products. J Clin Dent 2017;28(2):32–8.
59. Hitz Lindenmuller I, Lambrecht JT. Oral care. Curr Probl Dermatol 2011;40: 107–15.
60. Rose AJ, Fischer SH, Paasche-Orlow MK. Beyond medication reconciliation: the correct medication list. JAMA 2017;317(20):2057–8.
61. Raphael S, Blinkhorn A. Is there a place for Tooth Mousse in the prevention and treatment of early dental caries? A systematic review. BMC Oral Health 2015; 15(1):113.
62. O'Mullane DM, Baez RJ, Jones S, et al. Fluoride and oral health. Community Dent Health 2016;33(2):69–99.
63. Kumar S, Tadakamadla J, Johnson NW. Effect of toothbrushing frequency on incidence and increment of dental caries: a systematic review and meta-analysis. J Dent Res 2016;95(11):1230–6.
64. Reeson MG, Jepson NJ. Customizing the size of toothbrush handles for patients with restricted hand and finger movement. J Prosthet Dent 2002; 87(6):700.
65. Yaacob M, Worthington HV, Deacon SA, et al. Powered versus manual toothbrushing for oral health. Cochrane Database Syst Rev 2014;(6):CD002281.
66. De Visschere LM, van der Putten GJ, Vanobbergen JN, et al, Dutch Association of Nursing Home Physicians. An oral health care guideline for institutionalised older people. Gerodontology 2011;28(4):307–10.
67. Papas AS, Singh M, Harrington D, et al. Reduction in caries rate among patients with xerostomia using a power toothbrush. Spec Care Dentist 2007;27(2): 46–51.

68. Weyant RJ, Tracy SL, Anselmo TT, et al. Topical fluoride for caries prevention: executive summary of the updated clinical recommendations and supporting systematic review. J Am Dent Assoc 2013;144(11):1279–91.
69. Crystal YO, Niederman R. Evidence-based dentistry update on silver diamine fluoride. Dent Clin North Am 2019;63(1):45–68.
70. Peng JJ, Botelho MG, Matinlinna JP. Silver compounds used in dentistry for caries management: a review. J Dent 2012;40(7):531–41.
71. Horst JA, Ellenikiotis H, Milgrom PL. UCSF protocol for caries arrest using silver diamine fluoride: rationale, indications and consent. J Calif Dent Assoc 2016; 44(1):16–28.
72. Oliveira BH, Cunha-Cruz J, Rajendra A, et al. Controlling caries in exposed root surfaces with silver diamine fluoride: a systematic review with meta-analysis. J Am Dent Assoc 2018;149(8):671–9.e1.
73. Hendre AD, Taylor GW, Chavez EM, et al. A systematic review of silver diamine fluoride: effectiveness and application in older adults. Gerodontology 2017; 34(4):411–9.
74. Crystal YO, Marghalani AA, Ureles SD, et al. Use of silver diamine fluoride for dental caries management in children and adolescents, including those with special health care needs. Pediatr Dent 2017;39(5):135–45.
75. Leslie W, Hankey C. Aging, nutritional status and health. Healthcare (Basel) 2015; 3(3):648–58.
76. Sheiham A, James WP. A reappraisal of the quantitative relationship between sugar intake and dental caries: the need for new criteria for developing goals for sugar intake. BMC Public Health 2014;14:863.
77. Bailey RL, Ledikwe JH, Smiciklas-Wright H, et al. Persistent oral health problems associated with comorbidity and impaired diet quality in older adults. J Am Diet Assoc 2004;104(8):1273–6.
78. Kaye EK, Heaton B, Sohn W, et al. The dietary approaches to stop hypertension diet and new and recurrent root caries events in men. J Am Geriatr Soc 2015; 63(9):1812–9.
79. Riley P, Moore D, Ahmed F, et al. Xylitol-containing products for preventing dental caries in children and adults. Cochrane Database Syst Rev 2015;(3):CD010743.
80. Walsh T, Oliveira-Neto JM, Moore D. Chlorhexidine treatment for the prevention of dental caries in children and adolescents. Cochrane Database Syst Rev 2015;(4):CD008457.
81. Papas AS, Vollmer WM, Gullion CM, et al. Efficacy of chlorhexidine varnish for the prevention of adult caries: a randomized trial. J Dent Res 2012;91(2): 150–5.
82. Schwendicke F, Frencken JE, Bjorndal L, et al. Managing carious lesions: consensus recommendations on carious tissue removal. Adv Dent Res 2016; 28(2):58–67.
83. Rasines Alcaraz MG, Veitz-Keenan A, Sahrmann P, et al. Direct composite resin fillings versus amalgam fillings for permanent or adult posterior teeth. Cochrane Database Syst Rev 2014;(3):CD005620.
84. Schwendicke F, Gostemeyer G, Blunck U, et al. Directly placed restorative materials: review and network meta-analysis. J Dent Res 2016;95(6):613–22.
85. Gregory D, Hyde S. Root caries in older adults. J Calif Dent Assoc 2015;43(8): 439–45.
86. Caplan DJ, Li Y, Wang W, et al. Dental restoration longevity among geriatric and special needs patients. JDR Clin Trans Res 2019;4(1):41–8.

87. da Mata C, Allen PF, McKenna G, et al. Two-year survival of ART restorations placed in elderly patients: a randomised controlled clinical trial. J Dent 2015; 43(4):405–11.
88. da Mata C, Allen PF, Cronin M, et al. Cost-effectiveness of ART restorations in elderly adults: a randomized clinical trial. Community Dent Oral Epidemiol 2014;42(1):79–87.
89. da Mata C, Cronin M, O'Mahony D, et al. Subjective impact of minimally invasive dentistry in the oral health of older patients. Clin Oral Investig 2015; 19(3):681–7.
90. Zimmerman S, Sloane PD, Cohen LW, et al. Changing the culture of mouth care: mouth care without a battle. Gerontologist 2014;54(Suppl 1):S25–34.

The Interprofessional Role in Dental Caries Management

Impact of the Nursing Profession in Early Childhood Caries

Judith Haber, PhD, APRN*, Erin Hartnett, DNP, PPCNP-BC, CPNP

KEYWORDS

• Caries • Caries management • Interprofessional • Nursing • Midwifery • Pediatric
• Oral health

KEY POINTS

• Early childhood caries is a major unmet population health care need that negatively affects the overall health of children.

• Children from diverse racial/ethnic background and disadvantaged socioeconomic groups are especially affected by early childhood caries.

• Interprofessional pediatric oral health policy, education, and practice initiatives that have challenged the status quo are discussed, including those exemplars specific to advancing integration of oral health into the education and clinical practice of nurses, nurse practitioners, and midwives.

• The nursing profession is well positioned to have a positive impact on children's oral health and, in so doing, their overall health.

Early childhood caries (ECC) is a major unmet population health care need that negatively affects the overall health of children, especially those from diverse racial/ethnic backgrounds and disadvantaged socioeconomic groups. In 2000, the Surgeon General's seminal report, *Oral Health in America*, asserted that ECC was a "silent epidemic" of significant proportions.[1] Yet, 5 times more common than asthma, ECC remains the most common chronic disease of childhood.[1] Oral health is one of the Healthy People 2020 (HP2020) leading health indicators. All of the HP2020 oral health goals have shown improvement except for the number of children and adolescents

Disclosure Statement: The authors have received funding from DentaQuest and Arcora Foundations and the name of the grant is The Oral Health Nursing Education and Practice (OHNEP) Program.
NYU Rory Meyers College of Nursing, 433 First Avenue, New York, NY 10010, USA
* Corresponding author.
E-mail address: jh33@nyu.edu

who see a dentist.[2] Data from 2015 to 2016 reveal that 43% of children ages 2 to 19 had cavities, which was down from 50% 4 years earlier[3]; the proportion of children from ages 3 to 5 and 6 to 9 years with experience of dental caries in at least one primary or permanent tooth has been reduced from 33% to 29.7% for ages 3 to 5 years and 54.4% to 51.7% for ages 6 to 9 years.[2] School-age children lose 34 million school hours annually as a consequence of oral health problems related to pain, infection, and disrupted sleep and attentiveness.[4] The social determinants also affect oral health; children from families with lower levels of education and low socioeconomic status as well as specific racial/ethnic minority groups have higher rates of ECC. For example, Hispanic children had the highest prevalence of cavities at 52%.[3]

Oral health has been a neglected but important component of pediatric overall health. The historic separation of the mouth from the body, education and clinical practice silos, a fee-for-service, and individual versus a population-focused health delivery system all contribute to the omission of oral health as a required component of clinical education and practice.[5–7]

There are 4 million registered nurses, including 270,000 nurse practitioners and 13,000 midwives, the largest component of the in the United States health care workforce.[8] Nurses and nurse practitioners who work with young children and their families, as well as nurses and midwives who work with pregnant women, have a unique opportunity to positively influence the oral health and overall health of this population. With appropriate education to build their knowledge base and clinical practice competencies, the nursing profession has a unique opportunity to have a major impact on improving children's access to oral care and influencing oral health and overall health outcomes of this population.

In the past decade, interprofessional organizations have challenged the belief that oral health is solely the domain of the dental profession. The American Academy of Pediatrics (AAP), American Academy of Pediatric Dentistry (AAPD), American Academy of Physician Assistants, and the Oral Health Nursing Education and Practice Program (OHNEP) have played an interprofessional leadership role in developing numerous education, practice, and regulatory policies and products aimed at increasing the oral health knowledge, practice behaviors, and reimbursement of non-dental providers, thereby decreasing barriers to oral health care for children.[9,10] Moreover, oral health primary prevention requires more workforce capacity than the dental community alone can provide. Development of interprofessional oral health primary care workforce capacity is integral to increasing access to oral health care for the most vulnerable populations: pregnant women, children, and the poor, elderly, and infirm. Improving children's oral health outcomes is a leading population health goal; however, curricula preparing pediatric health professionals have had a dearth of oral health content and clinical experiences. The nursing profession now plays a leadership role in addressing the oral health needs of vulnerable populations across the lifespan, most notably children, their families, and communities.

PREGNANCY

Evidence supports that lack of oral health care during pregnancy is associated with negative outcomes for both mothers and their newborns. Building interprofessional oral health workforce capacity is integral to improving the overall health outcomes for mothers and babies.[11] During pregnancy, a woman's oral health can affect her health and the health of her unborn child. Nurses, nurse practitioners, and midwives are essential health care providers who can recognize and prevent many oral health problems during pregnancy.[11–13] Nurses, while caring for pregnant women, can use the Oral Health Delivery Framework (**Box 1**) as a model for integrating oral health in clinical encounters. They also can use the HEENOT approach when conducting the health history and physical examination. The HEENOT approach includes assessing the head, ears, eyes, nose, lips, mucous membranes, teeth, gums, and tongue rather than only the head, ears, eyes, nose, and throat (HEENT).[14] Prevention of oral health problems during pregnancy includes dispelling myths about the dangers of dental care during pregnancy. It includes information about oral hygiene, such as the importance of regular brushing twice a day and flossing daily. Preventing enamel erosion in women who experience pregnancy-induced vomiting includes instructing women to rinse with a solution of baking soda after vomiting.[11,15] Mothers need to know that if they have dental caries, *Streptococcus mutans*, the bacteria associated with dental caries, can be transmitted to their child, infect the child's teeth, and increase the risk for ECC.[11,16,17]

An example of the oral health impact of nurses during pregnancy is provided by a 2015 to 2016 pilot program with the Nurse Family Partnership (NFP), a nationwide home-visiting program of nurses assigned to first-time at-risk mothers. These nurses visit a pregnant woman throughout her pregnancy and continue until the child is aged 2 years. The NFP nurse provides the mother with education, support, and guidance throughout her pregnancy and the child's early development and care. The 2015 to 2016 pilot program, led by the OHNEP team, trained 32 NFP nurse home visitors in Florida to implement the Cavity Free Kids (CFK) oral health curriculum.[18] The nurse home visitors were asked to use the CFK oral health curriculum during their home visits with first-time pregnant women and first-time mothers of children ages 0 to 2. Data from surveys were collected at 3 points in time (baseline, 30 days after implementing CFK education, and 90 days after implementing CFK education) from nurses and home-visit clients to measure improvements in their oral health knowledge and practices. Survey findings reveal that the NFP nurses increased integration of oral health into 100% of their visits for both pregnant women and their young children. The survey also showed a significant increase ($P<.05$) in the amount of oral health information clients reported receiving, as well as a significant increase ($P<.05$) in the number of mothers cleaning their child's mouth twice a day. The most rewarding response was that of the 10 children graduating at the Two Year NFP Program Graduation Ceremony, none had any white or brown spots on their teeth. The long-term goal is that this program will be integrated into the National NFP education program.

Since 2011, the OHNEP program has collaborated with the American College of Nurse Midwives (ACNM) to advance integration of oral health in midwifery education and practice, thereby strengthening interprofessional oral health midwifery workforce

---

Box 1
Oral health delivery framework for integrating oral health in clinical encounters

- *ASK* questions about oral health when completing the health history

- *LOOK* in the mouth and complete the intraoral examination

- *DECIDE* on the patient's risk factors and formulate your management plan including those related to the patient's oral health

- *ACT* to engage the patient in preventive interventions that include oral health (eg, motivational interviewing for lifestyle change, oral hygiene coaching, dental referrals)

- *DOCUMENT* oral health findings for the history, physical examination, risk factors, and interventions, including referrals

capacity to address this population health issue by sponsoring workshops and symposia at ACNM meetings, conducting webinars, disseminating publications, and cultivating oral health champions among midwifery leaders. These strategies have increased the visibility of oral health as an essential component of whole-person midwifery care. The latest editions of 4 required midwifery program textbooks now feature a chapter on oral health and pregnancy.[19-22] Oral health test items are included on the Midwifery Comprehensive Examination. According to the findings of a recent national survey, 33 of 39 (84%) midwifery programs in the United States report including oral health topics and/or clinical experiences in their curriculum.[23]

PEDIATRIC PRIMARY AND ACUTE CARE

The pediatric nursing workforce, that is, nurses and nurse practitioners who work with children from infancy through adolescence, can be prepared in their undergraduate or graduate education or through clinical professional development programs to integrate oral health competencies as a standard component of their scope of practice. Nursing interventions to reduce the incidence of ECC can be woven into existing pediatric primary and acute care. Integration should begin during the mother's pregnancy during antepartum visits when the mother's oral health status and its influence on her child can be woven into antepartum visits by the nurse or midwife, especially for high-risk populations. It can also be highlighted by the newborn nursery nurse providing information to parents about the oral health care of their newborn during their postpartum stay in the hospital or birthing center. For example, an oral health education program for new mothers at a public hospital in an urban setting was devised[24] to determine the mothers' knowledge base about the oral health of newborns and young infants and assess the effectiveness of an oral health education program viewed before the mother's discharge from the postpartum unit. New mothers (n = 94) either viewed an evidence-based DVD about oral health care of their newborns or a DVD on newborn nutrition. Baseline data on a pretest revealed a significant lack of knowledge related to the need for infants' gums or teeth to be cleaned following eating or drinking (P<.02), and a significant number of mothers in the oral health education group responded yes (P<.01) about the benefits of fluoride varnish in ECC prevention. High attrition related to the transient nature of the study population was associated with low mother-infant response at 6- and 12-month follow-up visits. However, of the 10 infants who did return from the oral health education group, there was no evidence of white spots or dental caries on any tooth surface in the 8 to 12 erupted teeth. Each of the mothers had established a dental home for her infant by 1 year of age, which is consistent with recommendations from the AAPD and the AAP.[24]

Pediatric primary care settings are ideal for integrating oral health into the overall health care of young children who have 12 well-child visits to their primary care provider team by age 3 years. The pediatric office-based nurse, nurse practitioner, and/or community health nurse is in a position to reinforce oral health information, including guidance during well-child or home visits, about establishing a dental home by age 1 year. For example, nurses can coach parents about food and drinks, including formula, milk, breast milk, and juice, that play an important role in the development of ECC in primary teeth. They can reinforce that infants are at greater risk for developing tooth decay in primary teeth when they fall asleep with breast milk, a bottle of formula, sweetened drinks, or sweetened pacifier on their gums and teeth. Also vulnerable are toddlers who walk around all day with a bottle or "Sippy" cup filled with soda or juice. They need to emphasize that promoting oral hygiene practices, beginning with cleaning the gums of newborns with a gauze or washcloth after feeding to supervised tooth brushing once the first teeth erupt, is essential for removing foods that stick to the teeth or are high in sugar content.[24]

School settings, starting with Day Care, Head Start, and Elementary Schools, are ideal locations for oral health screenings, cariogenic nutrition education, fluoride varnish, and sealant applications. From 2012 to 2015, the Los Angeles Trust for Children's Health developed a school-based oral health program that established a District Oral Health Nurse position to coordinate oral health services, and implemented a universal school-based oral health screening and fluoride varnishing program, with referral to a dental home. School nurses implemented the parent, staff, and student education as well as the referrals and collaboration with community dental partners who did the screening and fluoride varnishing.[25] The program had a positive impact on reducing tooth decay in school-age children. Outcome data from 2015 to 2016 reveal that for 6 elementary schools with 3 dental provider groups, 491 parents received oral health education and 89 parents served as community volunteers. For this sample, 3399 screenings and 2776 fluoride varnish applications were completed. Sixty-six percent of the children had active disease, 27% had visible tooth decay, and 6% required emergent care. Of the 623 children who participated for 2 consecutive years, 56% had fewer or no visible caries at follow-up. Only 17% had additional disease. The annual cost was $69.57 per child, less than the cost of one cavity restoration.[25]

Pediatric nurse practitioners at New York University (NYU) Rory Meyers College of Nursing collaborate with NYU dental students on outreach to Head Start centers where they learn and practice the oral examination and fluoride varnish application with dental students; they assist the dental students to learn about and practice behavior management of children. The nursing profession is well positioned to have a positive impact on children's oral health and, in so doing, their overall health.

To encourage both interprofessional collaboration and oral health education, NYU College of Nursing, College of Dentistry, and School of Medicine have developed an interprofessional pediatric oral health experience as part of the College of Nursing's Teaching Oral Systemic Health program funded through an Advanced Nursing Education grant from the Health Resources and Services Administration (HRSA).[26] The clinical experience consists of teams of NYU nurse practitioner, MD, and dental surgery doctorate students, working together with a trained pediatric dental resident facilitator in the pediatric dental clinic and pediatric primary care clinic during a 4-hour clinical session to develop both oral health and interprofessional competencies. Students complete a pre– and post–Interprofessional Collaborative Competency Attainment Survey (ICCAS), which is a 20-item Likert scale based on self-reported interprofessional competencies. Data from the pre- and post-ICCAS demonstrate a significant increase in self-reported interprofessional competencies from pre to post experience for students across all 3 types and all 6 competencies. Survey data from 2015 to 2016 reveal that all students had an improved mean score from pretest to post-test after the experience, and these changes were statistically significant for all students: College of Nursing ($P<.01$), College of Dentistry ($P<.01$), and School of Medicine ($P<.001$). The mean change from pretest to post-test was statistically significant for each of the 6 interprofessional competency domains ($P<.01$) and in both pediatric dental and primary care settings, the changes from pre to post were significant ($P<.001$). These findings suggest that a clinical approach is an effective strategy for influencing the development of interprofessional and oral health competencies in all students.[26]

It is important to consider that not all children are attending school or having pediatric well visits because of either serious acute or chronic illness, and may not be accessing routine preventive dental care. Children being treated for cancer are at high risk for oral health problems, yet preventive dental care is not usually a priority during this time. Early assessment can identify oral complications of cancer treatment, and oral health intervention can reduce the severity of oral soft-tissue disorders, mucositis, and/or fungal infections or dental caries. To address this serious problem, advanced practice nurses, registered nurses, and oncology providers at the Stephen D. Hassenfeld Children's Center for Cancer and Blood Disorders, part of Hassenfeld Children's Hospital at NYU Langone, and the NYU College of Dentistry have been collaborating in an oral health program since 2011. The program, Chemo Without Cavities, has become a practice standard that integrates oral assessment and fluoride varnish into the care of all pediatric oncology patients.[27] All pediatric oncology patients, whether inpatient or outpatient, are screened by a pediatric dental resident before treatment begins, continuous oral assessment throughout treatment occurs at each visit by an interprofessional team of nurse practitioners, registered nurses, MDs, and pediatric dental residents, and each patient receives fluoride varnishing every 3 months. Patients are assured immediate access to dental care, if needed, by the NYU College of Dentistry.[27]

INTERPROFESSIONAL PEDIATRIC ORAL HEALTH EDUCATION RESOURCES

There are many open-access resources to promote oral health education in nursing education and practice. The OHNEP program has developed an Interprofessional Oral Health Faculty Toolkit, an innovative, Web-based, open-source product intended to facilitate the integration of oral-systemic health content and clinical competencies into nurse practitioner and midwifery curricula, which is based on the Interprofessional Education and Practice Competencies (2016), the National Organization of Nurse Practitioner Faculties Core Competencies (2017), and the HRSA (2014) interprofessional oral health core competencies delineated in the Integration of Oral Health and Primary Care Practice report (2014).[28–30] The Interprofessional Oral Health Faculty Toolkit is organized by program and describes how to "weave" evidence-based oral-systemic health content, teaching-learning strategies, and clinical experiences into pediatric, family, adult-gerontology, acute care, women's health, psychiatric-mental health nurse practitioner, and midwifery programs. The Pediatric and Midwifery Interprofessional Oral Health Faculty Toolkits can serve as a starting point for faculty, clinicians, and organizations as they work to play a leadership role in building interprofessional oral health workforce capacity to improve oral health access, decrease oral health disparities, improve oral health and overall health outcomes, prepare for accreditation, and enhance the health of the communities they serve.[31] This Toolkit uses the HEENOT approach previously described.[14] It includes a wealth of oral-systemic health resources for health assessment, health promotion, and clinical practice for faculty, students, and practicing clinicians to teach both the theory and practice of the integration of oral health into the history and physical examination. Examples of the Toolkit's overall strategies include (1) visual aids to supplement class discussions of normal versus abnormal oral findings, (2) oral-systemic case studies, and (3) projects to develop oral health education resources. It also provides specific strategies to teach future providers how to promote effective self-management of oral and overall health in their patients through interprofessional collaborative practice, health literacy, and community service.[31]

Another online resource has been developed by the National League for Nursing (NLN), a Web-based series about Advancing Care Excellence in Pediatrics (ACE.P). With generous funding from the Hearst Foundation, the unfolding ACE.P cases highlight the impact of the social determinants of health on access to care for children in vulnerable populations. The cases focus on the special needs of vulnerable children in the areas of nutrition/obesity, oral health, preventive care, immunizations, mental health, and autism. The ACE.P cases follow the format of NLN's highly regarded and successful Advancing Care Excellence for Vulnerable Populations (ACE) series.[32]

For example, the ACE.P presents an unfolding oral health case in 3 different scenarios: first, in an outpatient pediatric clinic when Mia Jones, a 4-year-old, comes in for immunizations and the nurse discovers she has ECC; the second scenario is 3 months later when Mia is recovering in the postanesthesia care unit after surgery for ECC; and 3 months later in the emergency department after Mia falls from the monkey bars and has dental trauma. These are all real pediatric oral health problems that nurses in pediatric care may experience and need the knowledge and skills to evaluate, educate, treat, and refer. ACE.P also presents teaching strategies for faculty to integrate this information into their curriculum.[32] The ACE.P program is a high-impact, open-access resource on the NLN Web site with potential exposure to 40,000 individual and 1200 organizational NLN faculty members.

RECOMMENDATIONS

The most important recommendation is to use the numerous nursing exemplars described in this article to weave into any existing pediatric primary or acute care educational or clinical program. The majority focuses on preventive assessment and interventions that can be used to reduce the incidence of ECC. For nursing, nurse practitioner, or midwifery students, integration should begin in their Health Assessment course and be woven throughout their undergraduate and graduate classroom content and clinical experiences. Results of students' surveys from the interprofessional pediatric oral health experience described earlier indicate effectiveness in developing interprofessional competencies using oral health as an exemplar. Integrating interprofessional oral health experiences in the nursing curriculum has been facilitated by the accreditation requirement that most health professional programs show evidence of exposing students to interprofessional classroom and/or clinical experiences in their curriculum. Interprofessional oral health experiences can include dental, dental hygiene, or dental assistant students as well as pharmacy, social work, nutrition, physical therapy, or speech therapy students. These experiences can be live or virtual. We also recommend cultivating one or more faculty or clinical oral health champions who support the integration of interprofessional oral health competencies and act as formal or informal leaders in advancing that agenda. Finally, we recommend increasing faculty commitment to standardizing integration of oral health content and clinical experiences across nursing program curricula through development of standardized oral health competencies. Developing relationships with colleagues in the dental and other professions is an excellent way to achieve that goal.

For nurses already in practice, we suggest that there are many examples of successful integration of oral care into existing practice: in schools, oncology centers, newborn nursery, and homecare. The NFP and pediatric oncology survey findings demonstrate the effectiveness of nurses in assessing and educating patients in oral health. The NFP, newborn nursery, and school health findings indicate positive patient outcomes when nurses educate mothers/caregivers in infant and child oral health. Nurses can work collaboratively to develop oral health programs within their existing practices by modifying workflow and oral health documentation requirements using interprofessional collaboration and teamwork.

SUMMARY

Oral health needs to be a standard component of nursing education and practice to address the oral health needs of populations across the lifespan. It is particularly important to address the links between oral health and overall health when caring for those who are most vulnerable and regardless of setting; namely, pregnant women, infants and children, and those with acute and chronic health problems. With appropriate oral health education and clinical competency development, the nursing profession is well positioned to have a positive impact on children's oral health and, in so doing, their overall health.

REFERENCES

1. US Department of Health and Human Services. Oral health in America: a report of the Surgeon General. Rockville (MD): U.S. Department of Health and Human Services, National Institute of Dental and Craniofacial Research, National Institutes of Health; 2000.
2. Healthy people 2020. Oral health of children and adolescents. In: 2020 topics & objectives: oral health. 2019. Available at: https://www.healthypeople.gov/2020/topics-objectives/topic/oral-health/objectives. Accessed January 29, 2019.
3. Centers for Disease Control and Prevention. Children's oral health. Available at: https://www.cdc.gov/OralHealth/children_adults/child.htm#1. Accessed January 30, 2019.
4. Naaval S, Kelekar U. School hours lost due to acute/unplanned dental care. Health Behav Policy Rev 2018;5(2):66–73.
5. Hummel J, Phillips KE, Holt B, et al. Oral health: an essential component of primary care. Seattle (WA): Qualis Health; 2015.
6. Institute of Medicine (IOM). Advancing oral health in America. Washington, DC: The National Academies Press; 2011.
7. Institute of Medicine (IOM), National Research Council (NRC). Improving access to oral health care for vulnerable and underserved populations. Washington, DC: The National Academies Press; 2011.
8. American Nurses Association (ANA). About ANA. Available at: https://www.nursingworld.org/ana/about-ana/. Accessed January 30, 2019.
9. Hallas DD, Shelley DD. Role of pediatric nurse practitioners in oral health care. Acad Pediatr 2009;9(6):462–6.
10. Hallas D, Fernandez JB, Herman NG, et al. Identification of pediatric oral health core competencies through interprofessional education and practice. Nurs Res Pract 2015;2015:360523.
11. Hartnett E, Haber J, Krainovich-Miller B, et al. Oral health in pregnancy. J Obstet Gynecol Neonatal Nurs 2016;45(4):565–73.
12. Kessler JL. A literature review on women's oral health across the life span. Nurs Womens Health 2017;21(2):108–21.
13. Oral Health Care During Pregnancy Expert Workgroup. Oral health care during pregnancy: a national consensus statement. Washington, DC: National Maternal and Child Oral Health Resource Center; 2012.
14. Haber J, Hartnett E, Hallas D, et al. Putting the mouth back in the head: HEENT to HEENOT. Am J Public Health 2015;105(3):437–41.
15. Silk H, Douglass AB, Douglass JM, et al. Oral health during pregnancy. Am Fam Physician 2008;77(8):1139–44.
16. Berkowitz RJ. Mutans streptococci: acquisition and transmission. Pediatr Dent 2006;28(2):106–9.

17. California Dental Association Foundation, American College of Obstetricians and Gynecologists District IX. Oral health during pregnancy and early childhood: evidence-based guidelines for health professionals. J Calif Dent Assoc 2010; 38:391–403, 405–40.

18. Hartnett E, Hille A. Teeth for two: oral health in pregnancy and early childhood. Presented at: National Oral Health Conference (NOHC), the 19th Annual Joint Meeting of the Association of State and Territorial Dental Directors (ASTDD) and the American Association of Public Health Dentistry (AAPHD). Louisville, KY, April 16–18, 2018.

19. King TL, Brucker MC, Osborne K, et al, editors. Varney's midwifery. 6th edition. Burlington (NJ): Jones & Bartlett Learning; 2019.

20. Hackley B, Kreibs J. Primary care of women. 2nd edition. Burlington (NJ): Jones & Bartlett Learning; 2017.

21. Tharpe NL, Farley CL, Jordan RG. Clinical practice guidelines for midwifery & women's health. 5th edition. Burlington (NJ): Jones & Bartlett Learning; 2017.

22. Kessler JL. Oral health. In: Jordan RG, Farley CL, Grace KT, editors. Prenatal and postnatal care: a woman-centered approach. 2nd edition. Hoboken (NJ): Wiley; 2019. p. 247–52.

23. Haber J, Dolce M, Hartnett E, et al. Integrating oral health curricula into midwifery graduate programs: results of a US survey. J Midwifery Womens Health 2019. https://doi.org/10.1111/jmwh.12974.

24. Hallas D, Fernandez JB, Lim JL, et al. OHEP: an oral health education program for mothers of newborns. J Pediatr Health Care 2015;29(2):181–90.

25. Dudovitz RN, Valiente JE, Espinosa G, et al. A school-based public health model to reduce oral health disparities. J Public Health Dent 2018;78:9–16.

26. Hartnett E, Haber J, Catapano P, et al. The impact of an interprofessional pediatric oral health clerkship on advancing interprofessional education outcomes. J Dent Educ 2019. https://doi.org/10.21815/JDE.019.088.

27. Hartnett E, Krainovich-Miller B. Preventive dental care: an educational program to integrate oral care into pediatric oncology. Clin J Oncol Nurs 2017;21(5):611–6.

28. Interprofessional Education Collaborative. Core competencies for interprofessional collaborative practice: 2016 update. Washington, DC: Interprofessional Education Collaborative; 2016.

29. NP Core Competencies Work Group, Curricular Leadership Committee. Nurse practitioner core competencies content. National Organization of Nurse Practitioner Faculties (NONPF). Available at: https://www.nonpf.org/page/14. Accessed January 31, 2019.

30. Health Resources and Services Administration. Integration of oral health and primary care practice report. Rockville (MD): U.S. Department of Health and Human Services; 2014.

31. Oral Health Nursing Education and Practice. Interprofessional oral health faculty toolkit for primary care nurse practitioner and midwifery programs. Available at: http://ohnep.org/faculty-toolkit. Accessed January 31, 2019.

32. National League for Nursing (NLN). ACE.P. Available at: http://www.nln.org/professional-development-programs/teaching-resources/ace-p. Accessed January 31, 2019.

The Interprofessional Role in Dental Caries Management
From the Social Worker Perspective

Kristen Flick, MSW[a],*, Leonardo Marchini, DDS, MSD, PhD[b]

KEYWORDS

- Social barriers in dentistry • Social worker in dentistry • Barriers to care

KEY POINTS

- Many people face barriers when pursuing dental care. Social workers are instrumental in connecting patients and families to resources that help to overcome these obstacles.
- Transportation is a common barrier in dental caries management. There are a variety of resources to assist with issues associated with transportation, including rides and gas reimbursement.
- Limited finances limit the dental care people can afford. Exploring local, state, and federal financial resources can help people to afford necessary dental care.
- Informed consent is essential in all dental treatment. Ensuring the legally appropriate person is consenting to treatment is particular important for minors and dependent adults.

Social workers are valuable members of any health care team, including oral health care. Social workers overcome challenges by connecting people to resources and assisting in the navigation of health care systems. Using the biopsychosocial perspective, social workers assist patients and families in overcoming barriers to care. This article outlines the most common obstacles for patients, including transportation, finances, and informed consent, as well as the enablers that help increase access to dental care. Special attention is paid to vulnerable populations and other types of social worker involvement.

Disclosure Statement: The authors have nothing to disclose.
[a] University of Iowa College of Dentistry and Dental Clinics, S345 DSB 801 Newton Road, Iowa City, IA 52242, USA; [b] Preventative and Community Dentistry, University of Iowa College of Dentistry and Dental Clinics, N3371 DSB 801 Newton Road, Iowa City, IA 52242, USA
* Corresponding author.
E-mail address: kristen-flick@uiowa.edu

BIOPSYCHOSOCIAL PERSPECTIVE

Social workers bring an important perspective to help engage patients in their oral health care. The biopsychosocial perspective explores the biological, psychological, and social aspects that affect patients and families every day, which allows social workers and others to identify and target the important factors that connect patients to oral health care. Biological factors may include physical health, genetic makeup, and oral anatomy. Psychological factors may include self-esteem and perceptions of dentists. Social factors may include family influence, school or work environment, and peer interactions. These factors all constantly interact for each individual, influencing people's relationships and personalities as well as their oral health care.

Considering the biological, psychological, and social facets of a person sheds light on the complexity of each individual as well as grants access to people's values and attitudes, which are important components of oral health.[1] Along with incorporating each person's values and attitudes, the biopsychosocial perspective blends well with the model of social determinants of health.[2] Factors commonly addressed in social work, including social support, culture, and socioeconomic status, affect outcomes in oral health for people across a variety of circumstances. Bearing in mind these concepts in oral health care is likely to increase access to oral health care needs and understanding of the patients being served. Examples of biopsychosocial factors are illustrated in **Fig. 1.**

BARRIERS

Exploring the complexity of each patient through the biopsychosocial model provides valuable insight into options to increase attendance at recall visits. The biopsychosocial model offers information on what else could be going on in a patient's

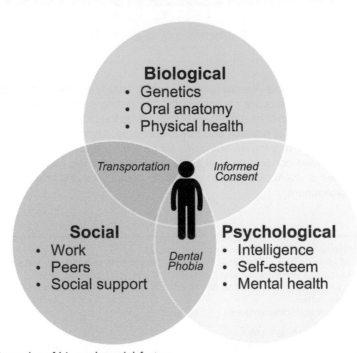

Fig. 1. Examples of biopsychosocial factors.

life that may be hindering him or her from attending a recall appointment. For example, priorities such as medical conditions, work schedule, or child rearing may be interfering with appointment attendance. Considering these factors and exploring solutions for the impeding barriers help providers better serve their patients and collaborate to develop an effective plan for recall appointments. Some of the most common barriers include transportation, finances, and informed consent.

Transportation

If patients cannot physically get to the dental office, it is particularly challenging for them to receive dental care. Transportation is a common barrier for patients, often due to cost or inability to drive. Many patients cannot drive themselves and must rely on someone else with a working vehicle and active driver's license to transport them to all appointments. These circumstances can be challenging for patients with limited social support and resources and is a time and financial commitment for the drivers. Other patients are able to drive, but do not have a reliable vehicle to get them to appointments, which may be a significant distance from their homes.

Many people cannot afford gas to travel to their dental appointments, especially when multiple visits are needed to complete treatment. In other circumstances, patients are required to pay for parking when visiting a dental office. These fees may cost more than the patient with limited finances is able to spare and thus deters people from seeking routine dental care.

Finances

Cost of treatment is a common consideration for many people seeking dental care. Paying for treatment out of pocket can be challenging and even impossible for many. Finances are especially relevant for those people with significant dental needs. Although dental insurance is a helpful option, it is not always a viable option. Some may not be able to afford the cost of dental insurance, and some plans do not cover the services that patients may be seeking. If patients cannot pay for dental treatment and do not have insurance, they may not pursue dental care until it reaches an emergency state. This delay provides time for more issues to manifest, particularly more severe consequences of dental caries.

Informed Consent

Providers have a legal and ethical responsibility to get informed consent for all procedures. If a patient cannot legally consent to his or her own treatment and does not bring the legal guardian to sign the treatment plan, he or she may not be able to pursue dental treatment. Minors and dependent adults cannot legally consent to their own dental treatment and must have a legal guardian or Power of Attorney (POA) present to consent to all treatment. A legal guardian is a person designated by a judge in a court of law who has the full decision-making rights of the ward. A POA may be established using a notary or lawyer and outlines which aspects of a person's life the POA is able to make decisions regarding, such as health care or finances. Informed consent is an essential component of any treatment completed, and ensuring the legally appropriate person is willing and able to consent can be a major obstacle for treatment.

Vulnerable Populations

Any pool of patients may experience barriers to dental care. However, there are certain groups that are more strongly impacted by these social obstacles, which negatively affect their oral health care. The most vulnerable populations include, but are not limited to, children, geriatric populations, those with low socioeconomic status, inmates, immigrants, refugees, and individuals with special needs. Transportation to appointments, paying for oral hygiene supplies, scheduling appointments, and meeting important dental needs are often especially challenging with these groups of patients, which could make the social worker's role even more valuable.

ENABLERS

There are many resources available to overcome these common barriers, and social workers often have regular interaction with these solutions. Working with an interdisciplinary team can help patients successfully overcome barriers to access and complete treatment.

Transportation

Transportation is a common barrier for a variety of patients, including low-income, elderly, and disabled people who have limited mobility and finances. Thankfully, many communities, organizations, and governments have included reliable, reasonable transportation resources in the resources they offer (**Box 1**). Some state-funded insurance plans pay for shuttle services to get low-income patients to appointments, or reimburse them for gas if they are able to drive themselves. Many churches and other nonprofit agencies offer assistance for costs or logistics of transportation, which can make all the difference in receiving dental care. Public transportation, when available, may provide a less expensive transportation option for those concerned with paying for a ride. All of these resources require some planning in advance to arrange the transportation services, but they are a reliable and sustainable option for many dental patients.

Finances

In focusing specifically on financial barriers, there are several avenues worth exploring by patients and dental providers in an effort to overcome financial obstacles (**Box 2**). The first is private dental insurance. Does the patient have it? What does it cover? Would the patient benefit from purchasing private dental insurance? Does the patient qualify for a less expensive insurance option, such as state dental insurance? These important questions help better understand the financial situations of those patients with private dental insurance, or those who would benefit from investing in private insurance.

For those patients who cannot afford private dental insurance, there may be helpful resources available through the state government. Applying for state dental insurance is free for the applicant and may provide insurance coverage at little or no cost to the member. It is commonly advised that patients apply for state insurance to see if they qualify, because there is no penalty for rejection, and the coverage, if accepted, is

---

Box 1
Transportation enablers

Shuttle provided by facility or insurance

Churches and nonprofit resources

Public transportation

Gas reimbursement

Assistance from family, friends, or nonprofit agencies

Box 2
Financial enablers
Private dental insurance
State dental insurance
Other state financial resources
Community action agencies
Assistance from churches or nonprofit agencies

quite helpful. Social workers often direct patients to this avenue if the patient meets the necessary income guidelines. Beyond state dental insurance, there may be other resources available to assist with the costs associated with dental treatment. Although each state differs in what they offer and the avenues to access it, social workers are valuable in directing patients to the resources that best fit their circumstances.

Beyond state resources, social workers are instrumental in exploring other assistance options. Oftentimes, community action agencies may help residents with heating assistance, transportation, child care, medical bills, and other needs. Some churches and nonprofit agencies have assistance options available as well. Exploring opportunities for other financial resources offers a creative way to decrease other financial burdens, thereby shifting patients' limited funds to contribute to oral health care.

Informed Consent

Informed consent is legally and ethically required before any treatment can be completed, which can be challenging for patients who are not their own medical decision maker. A legal guardian for a minor is the child's biological or adoptive parent, or another person designated as medical decision maker by a judge in a court of law. Foster parents, grandparents, and others do not receive these rights unless permitted by a judge. Getting informed consents can be especially challenging if the children do not live with their legal guardians, if the legal guardian is incarcerated, or if their whereabouts are unknown. For a dependent adult, a legal guardian or POA is accepted for medical decision making. It is advisable to review these documents carefully in order to understand the stipulations and to attach it to the patient's chart in case a question regarding consenting practices arises. Human services offices are often involved in these cases in making sure that the dependent persons receive necessary medical and dental care.

Vulnerable Populations

Social workers can help members of these groups access dental care by connecting them to resources, such as state or federal insurance applications, transportation options, and education. Coordinating care with other medical needs may also be a way to overcome some of the barriers hindering these groups from getting their oral health care needs met. If there are language, cognitive, or other barriers that are preventing patients from exploring these resources, social workers can be valuable in overcoming obstacles to connect patients to assistance options. Continually, forms of prejudice, such as ageism, may be addressed by social workers by providing support and advocacy. Advocates may strengthen patients' confidence in themselves and in the system, which will result in positive oral health care results. The smoother the process, the more likely people are to follow through.

SUMMARY

Networking with the social services resources within organizations and communities can help dental providers to better reach and serve their patient pool, which has positive implications for providers and patients alike. Awareness of where these resources may be found and what they offer is an important tool in serving a diverse patient pool. Social workers also consider the cultures and values of people. These cultures and values affect oral health care practices as well as perceptions of dental providers and treatment options and is a valuable part of gaining patients' compliance in oral health care.

Social workers play an important role in engaging patients in their oral health care. Understanding a holistic view of the person through a biopsychosocial model, connecting patients to resources, and paying special attention to the most vulnerable populations are some of the important pieces social workers contribute to the oral health treatment process. Social workers devote time to staying current on the evolving resources available, assisting patients in finding helpful tools for their care. Involving social workers in the coordination of care and caries management has the potential to improve outcomes and make the processes smoother for every member of the team.

REFERENCES

1. Glick M, Williams DM, Kleinman DV, et al. A new definition for oral health developed by the FDI World Dental Federation opens the door to a universal definition of oral health. Am J Orthod Dentofacial Orthop 2017;151(2):229–31.
2. Fisher-Owens SA, Gansky SA, Platt LJ, et al. Influences on children's oral health: a conceptual model. Pediatrics 2007;120(3):e510–20.

The Interprofessional Role in Dental Caries Management
Ways Medical Providers Can Support Oral Health (Perspectives from a Physician)

Susan A. Fisher-Owens, MD, MPH[a,b,*]

KEYWORDS

• Oral health • Dental caries • Interprofessional care • Medical care

KEY POINTS

• Medical providers play an important role counselling families on how to establish and keep healthy habits for a healthy mouth. By reaching families before a problem has started, medical providers can help stem the epidemic of oral disease.

• Fluoride varnish is a distinct modality to prevent childhood caries, which can and should be integrated into primary care.

• Referrals to a dental home should be made by the first birthday; medical providers should follow-up with these referrals as they would with any other, to insure patients are receiving this important care.

• Advocacy is a venue both to improve patients health and to increase interprofessional collaboration.

• Collaboration facilitates interprofessional relationships, which can help with urgent referrals or simply education. Such collaboration benefits the patient as well as the professionals' job satisfaction.

INTRODUCTION

Dentistry first was extracted from medical care in the seventeenth century and then excluded from medical school curricula in 1840. The first dental school was founded in the United States. Since then, many in allopathic medicine do not understand the

Disclosure Statement: The author has nothing to disclose.
[a] Department of Pediatrics, School of Medicine, University of California, San Francisco, San Francisco, CA, USA; [b] Department of Preventive and Restorative Dental Sciences, School of Dentistry, University of California, San Francisco, San Francisco, CA, USA
* Zuckerberg San Francisco General Hospital, 1001 Potrero Avenue/MS6D37, San Francisco, CA 94110.
E-mail address: Susan.Fisher-Owens@UCSF.edu

impact of oral disease on individuals, and the impact of oral disease exacerbating systemic health issues. However, an increasing percentage of medical providers recognize the impact of oral disease on systemic disease and the need to prevent disease where patients are seen, in the primary care medical office, ideally before they get sick. The workflow is not difficult to accommodate: oral health easily can be incorporated into risk assessment and physical examination. Counseling around preventing oral disease naturally builds off of current anticipatory guidance. With the recommendation of the US Preventive Services Task Force to have fluoride varnish applied at well child visits, there is even a mechanism to prevent or reverse early decay in the medical office, all while working to improve referrals to establish a patient in a dental home.

There are many ways different workforce can lend to improving access to oral health care. Some are discussed elsewhere in this issue. This article focuses on dental caries prevention and management in the medical home.

ROLES THROUGH THE AGES

To ask where oral health is first seen in the medical world is not a far cry from the old adage about the chicken and the egg. For the purpose of this discussion, we start with pediatrics, and then follow with obstetrics, internal medicine, and geriatrics.

Pediatrics

The natural first intersection between oral and systemic health is in the child's medical home. Of children who see medical and dental professionals, almost all see the medical provider, and see them first and more frequently. However, only 50% of all children 2 to 17 years saw a dentist in 2011[1]; in 2009, the rate was less than 8% for children younger than 3 years.[2] These facts establish the medical home as a valuable option for initial oral health education.

One of the best examples of oral health integration into pediatric primary care is Into the Mouths of Babes, in North Carolina,[3,4] with a sophisticated and thorough approach to integrating oral health. However, medical clinics without those resources[5] can still play an important role in children's oral health promotion.

Just like medical providers write their clinical documentation as a "SOAP note" (subjective/objective/assessment/plan), oral health can be integrated into the workflow using the SOAP structure. The subjective part of the note is when one is asking about patients' concerns, risky and preventive actions and behaviors, and personal and family history. Oral health risk assessments are a natural part of this process, and often the relevant screening questions are already being asked (eg, screening for obesity risk factors). Dental caries risk assessments can be incorporated into medical visits workflows, which then can help prioritize the provider's response[6–8] (see also National Network for Oral Health Access Oral Health Infrastructure toolkit, http://www.nnoha.org/ohi-toolkit/ohi-toolkit-background/).

Because of the great overlap between root causes of disease relating to social disparities/social determinants of health, including access to care, healthy activities, and nutritious foods, the medical profession serves patients by screening for adverse childhood experiences and other social determinants of health, and providing related support. Examples of such services include the medical legal partnership to help address legal concerns, housing referrals to address housing instability, or food prescriptions/food pantries in the clinic. These interventions all facilitate resolution of concerns more basic on Maslow's hierarchy of need, which only after they have been addressed will free families up to focus on important health initiatives.

Medical providers have a more specific role to support oral health. Understanding the family's health provides insight into an individual child's risk for oral health problems, and may open the discussion of dental anxiety, if any, or simply the self-efficacy about being able to prevent dental disease and pain.

The objective part of the medical evaluation is the physical examination, which should include the mouth, the teeth, and gums. The assessment and plan portion of the SOAP is the diagnoses and plan. The latter arguably is where the primary care provider can have greatest influence, by providing education, referrals, preventive services, and even treatments. Still, recognizing the issue and discussing it with the patient/family is key to moving to intervention and treatment.

Education

One could argue that the biggest role the pediatrician plays is introducing and then underscoring the importance of oral health. Teachable moments begin even before the first tooth has erupted. Guiding parents to see ways to soothe a baby that does not include food help with overall health in coming years. Similarly, getting the family to stop nighttime feeds (once appropriate) is better for the health of the teeth and mental health for the parents, and for the sleep routine for all. Perhaps most important is to encourage the family to pursue their own oral health, along with teaching about oral disease as an infectious disease that is spread vertically (mother to baby in utero, or after birth by caregiver to child) or horizontally (sibling to sibling, or baby to baby in a day care setting). This is particularly relevant when a child drops her pacifier on the ground, and the parent "cleans" it in his or her mouth instead of washing it off with water. This is a great opportunity to start discussing oral health, its role in systemic health, and the role of parents and patients in keeping healthy from the start or returning to full health as soon as possible.

Another educational program that can be shared out of the medical office is "Brush Book Bed." This program, introduced by the American Academy of Pediatrics, extends the work of "Reach Out and Read" by having pediatricians give a toothbrush along with a book at well-child visits. Educational materials are available for the office encouraging families to establish a nighttime routine of brushing the teeth, reading a book, and going to bed. Pilot studies on this intervention found families brushed the child's teeth more regularly, were more willing to go to a dentist, and liked the improved sleep hygiene for the child.

Another important role of primary care is that of making referrals to dental providers. Medical providers should refer to dental providers. Even as far back as 2004, dela Cruz and colleagues[9] found that almost 80% of providers would refer patients with signs of early decay or having high risk for future disease. Medical colleagues underscore the importance of oral health when making a referral for dental care and treating it like other referrals, providing information and following up that it happened. A patient is more likely to go to a dental provider if they are referred by a medical provider, whether from pediatrics,[10] obstetrics,[11,12] or other fields. Assistance to providers in referrals, such as by community health workers, can increase the proportion of patients who arrive to a dental visit.[13]

Since placing referrals has been insufficient to see epidemiology for this disease drop, it is important that medical professionals add prevention into their arsenal for fighting oral disease.

Prevention

Pediatricians have long been responsible for prescribing fluoride tablets in the setting of a patient who does not have access to adequately fluoridated water. Still, a prescription is insufficient to provide optimal oral health care. Beyond just mentioning the importance of starting tooth-brushing, with fluoridated toothpaste as soon as the first tooth erupts, pediatricians should be prepared to counsel on oral health issues. Moreover, they often are approached with questions around behavior issues, such as children refusing to brush. Therefore, responses are facilitated by an understanding of oral health and development.

Moreover, medical teams can counsel about tobacco use (for the parent or the child) and prescribe antibiotic prophylaxis (or antianxiety medications) as needed before patient visits.

A tangible way to support patients' prevention is fluoride varnish. This prophylaxis has been used in the medical setting for more than a decade, as a way to help prevent oral health problems until that time when a child is established into a dental home. It is applied twice a year and decreases the risk of dental decay in primary teeth by 37%,[14] and is effective in reversing up to 64% of decay.[15]

Treatment

If dental caries is allowed to progress, it turns into a soft tissue infection which can further progress to life-threatening disease. It is imperative that medical providers (particularly those in the emergency department and those caring for children in general) are able to start appropriate antibiotic therapy, and then facilitate the child being seen by a dentist posthaste.

Silver diamine fluoride is another combined preventive and treatment tool that has been used in nontraumatic dental care. Medical providers around the country who live in low-access areas have started to apply silver diamine fluoride as a way to stop current and prevent further delay. Use of this intervention in the medical home is in its nascency. Still, it is important for medical providers to be aware of which dental providers in their community use this modality, to help educate families about this non-invasive intervention as an option that does not require sedation, and to refer accordingly, as well as not to be surprised if seeing the darkened, treated lesions during an exam.

Obstetrics

Pregnancy is a seminal moment in a woman's life, when she often is more motivated than ever to improve her health status, even if just as a way of helping her baby. Moreover, pregnancy is a time when women may have access to care by having dental insurance coverage, which they do not normally have. It is completely safe to provide care to women during pregnancy, and some research has shown improvements with low birth weight, premature birth, and stillbirth.[16–23]

The subjective questions are in the same realm as with pediatrics, but with the important caveat that pregnancy can cause additional risks, such as hyperemesis, with the impact of acid on the teeth, or even simple morning sickness, which often leads women to increase the frequency of their simple carbohydrate snacking, and thus influences the pH of the mouth and resulting increased caries formation.

Objectively, providers should be aware of and examine women for pregnancy granulomas and pregnancy gingivitis.

When reviewing the assessment and plan with a pregnant woman, it is an opportune time to reiterate the importance of oral habits because the woman is "brushing for two."[24] In addition, establishing good habits at this point can help set the foundation for the mother to provide quality infant oral health care. Referrals are particularly important for women when pregnant, for several reasons. Pragmatically, women who may not have coverage at other times in their life do during pregnancy, so it is important to capitalize on these services. Also, because women are at higher risk for oral health complications during pregnancy, it is important for medical providers to be aware of these conditions, so they can assist and refer appropriately.

Harborview Medical Center is an example of a facility integrating oral health with prenatal care, through patient education starting with the first prenatal visit.[25]

Internal Medicine

A basic fact for adults is that regular health insurance does not include dental insurance. In 2017, more than 27 million Americans did not have health insurance,[26] less than half the population that did not have dental insurance at the same time, approximately 74 million (~23%).[26,27] Even the Affordable Care Act did not include dental insurance as an essential and mandatory benefit (effectively saying that it was important, but would not involve a penalty if patients did not sign up for it). Thus, many adults have at baseline a decreased access to care.

However, increasingly literature is coming out about the role of oral health in systemic health. A prime example of this is with diabetes, a condition affecting more than 9% of the adult population and responsible for some of the greatest burden of disease.[28] It is imperative that patients with diabetes be referred for regular oral health care. Research has shown that preventive periodontal care may decrease cost of overall medical care.[29] Other conditions with strong systemic and dental illness include cardiovascular disease,[30,31] pneumonia,[32] end-stage renal disease,[33,34] and stroke.[35]

Great examples of integrated medical-dental care in the United States are Kaiser Permanente's Eugene Oregon clinic and the Marshfield Clinic in Wisconsin.[36,37]

Emergency Department

Nationally, the rates of visits in the emergency room for oral health problems is increasing.[38] There is a major burden on the health care system of patients visiting the emergency department for nontraumatic dental pain, in terms of people and of dollars (estimated 1.6 billion).[38] Emergency providers play an important role in stabilizing the patient's pain and referring them to appropriate care.

Geriatrics

Patients in their golden years may not be receiving platinum oral health care. There is a particular challenge with getting patients from nursing homes to dental providers which is a fundamental access barrier. Expansion of care through registered dental hygienists in alternative practice and dental therapists may help lessen the load requirement of dentists by improving access to preventive care and basic treatment.

Medically, research reports the link between poor oral health and increase in systemic health issues. Medical providers must mention the need for continued oral health care (and not support the fatalism of "they're going to fall out anyway" similar to the unconcern associated with ignorance about importance of keeping baby teeth healthy) and help prioritize this care for patients, particularly when they have multiple medical concerns, many of which are impacted by poor oral health. These include being more likely to develop[39–42] and have more rapid cognitive decline with dementia, and more likely to have incidents/accidents in addition to the health conditions above.[43,44]

Location

Thus, there are many ways medical professionals can support oral health care by offering education, referral, preventive services, and some treatment. There are also multiple models of how a medical home can integrate oral health.

The natural way medical providers deal with issues that they think are outside of their scope is with referrals. Many medical providers start by making referrals to oral health providers. Although this does increase the likelihood of a patient going to a dentist relative to if nothing is done, it has been ineffective to solve the oral health crisis.

Colocation is a significant but insufficient next step. For instance, even at federally qualified health centers (FQHCs) where medical and dental are colocated, fewer than 40% of patients regularly are seen in both settings (Hilton, personal communication, 2016).

Coscheduling, when dental appointments are scheduled from the medical office, is a further step at improving dental referral rates. Few electronic health records have the capacity to do this, but it would reduce barriers to making appointments. The Marshfield Clinic in Wisconsin is one example that does have an integrated electronic medical-dental record, and better metrics of care.

For in-clinic care, different pilots have taken place around the country, with having a dental hygienist[45,46] or even a dentist[47] spend some or full time in clinic, providing dental services in the medical care visit.

Last, medical and dental offices can work together in overseeing outreach activities, to provide a more holistic set of services.

ROLES WITH DIFFERENT STAGES OF PROFESSIONALS
Pregraduate

The first step in facilitating medical professionals' role in oral health is to add to the education of premedical students. Although dentists know this fundamentally, it shocks medical professionals to be told that dental caries is the most common chronic disease of childhood. A decade ago, 70% of medical schools responding to a study reported having fewer than 5 hours of oral health curriculum, and 10% taught no coursework on oral health.[48]

Now, interprofessional training is offered at 90% of medical schools, and Harvard is offering extended training for practitioners trained in oral health and primary care.

Postgraduate

Because of the increase in schools providing interprofessional training over the past decade, there may be more of a need to educate postgraduate medical providers who have been out for longer as compared with recent graduates. Medical providers can play an additional, important role in supporting oral health. Any effort to break down silos is important, particularly when all are working separately to promote health overall. Moreover, there is a lot to learn from one another. As increasing numbers of medical schools are offering oral health education, more interaction, but for practitioners already in the field, working together for education can increase collaboration. Dental providers will find motivational interviewing, a technique that can be taught by medical providers, helpful to facilitate patient change; pediatric providers also can consult general dentists on how to work with young children. Meanwhile, dental providers can teach medical providers about oral health.

When medical and dental providers cross-train, they benefit not only from the information shared but also from building interprofessional relationships, which can help facilitate care or provide "curbside" consultations.

ADVOCACY

A related, and also mutually beneficial, activity is for medical and dental providers to collaborate on advocacy projects. Advocacy is an important intersection of the professions, and it can help each to get the other's professional body to support certain causes. First, when dental providers alone lobby for increased reimbursement, such as from Medicaid/Dentacaid and Medicare, they are seen as self-interested, but when medical providers speak on behalf of the importance of adequate dental reimbursement, the request is viewed more objectively. This is similarly true with funding research for oral health. Other topics that seem to be natural areas for joint advocacy are around workforce issues, policies requiring screening without treatment, availability of dental services in FQHCs, community water fluoridation, state child health insurance program (SCHIP [State Children's Health Insurance Program]), dental, WIC benefits (particularly for getting juice removed), school nutrition, and other nutrition including sugar-sweetened beverages. Collaborating on advocacy projects has the additional benefit of building interprofessional relationships, which can help on the clinical side when a pressing clinical question or referral arises. The first step toward this end may be as simple as compiling a referral list for one's local area, if it does not already exist.

SUMMARY

There are many ways that medical providers can promote oral health. Through counseling in clinic, encouraging referrals, and even applying preventive fluoride, medical providers can directly and positively impact oral health. By collaborating on advocacy efforts, medical and dental providers can improve their local and broader relationships with the end goal of improved health for patients throughout their lifetime.

REFERENCES

1. Soni, Anita. Children's Dental Care: Advice and Checkups, Ages 2–17, 2008. Statistical Brief #326. June 2011. Rockville (MD): Agency for Healthcare Research and Quality. Available at: http://www.meps.ahrq.gov/mepsweb/data_files/publications/st326/stat326.pdf.
2. Griffin SO, Barker LK, Wei L, et al. Use of dental care and effective preventive services in preventing tooth decay among U.S. Children and adolescents–Medical Expenditure Panel Survey, United States, 2003-2009 and National Health and Nutrition Examination Survey, United States, 2005-2010. MMWR Surveill Summ 2014;63(Suppl 2):54–60.
3. Rozier RG, Sutton BK, Bawden JW, et al. Prevention of early childhood caries in North Carolina medical practices: implications for research and practice. J Dent Educ 2003;67(8):876–85.
4. Stearns SC, Rozier RG, Kranz AM, et al. Cost-effectiveness of preventive oral health care in medical offices for young Medicaid enrollees. Arch Pediatr Adolesc Med 2012;166(10):945–51.
5. Atchison KA, Weintraub JA, Rozier RG. Bridging the dental-medical divide: case studies integrating oral health care and primary health care. J Am Dent Assoc 2018;149(10):850–8.
6. HRSA, Integration of oral health and primary care practice. 2014. p. 21.
7. American Academy of Pediatrics Section on Oral Health. Maintaining and improving the oral health of young children. Pediatrics 2014;134(6):1224–9.
8. Caries-risk assessment and management for infants, children, and adolescents. Pediatr Dent 2017;39(6):197–204.
9. dela Cruz GG, Rozier RG, Slade G. Dental screening and referral of young children by pediatric primary care providers. Pediatrics 2004;114(5):e642–52.
10. Beil HA, Rozier RG. Primary health care providers' advice for a dental checkup and dental use in children. Pediatrics 2010;126(2):e435–41.

11. Rocha JS, Arima LY, Werneck RI, et al. Determinants of dental care attendance during pregnancy: a systematic review. Caries Res 2018;52(1–2):139–52.
12. Corchuelo-Ojeda J, Perez GJ. Socioeconomic determinants of dental care during pregnancy in Cali, Colombia. Cad Saude Publica 2014;30(10):2209–18 [in Spanish].
13. Fontana M, Wallace R, Girdwood J, et al. Impact of a community health worker on interprofessional caries referrals (Abstract at 66th ORCA Congress, Cartagena, Colombia). Caries Res 2019;53:357–410.
14. Marinho VC, Worthington HV, Walsh T, et al. Fluoride varnishes for preventing dental caries in children and adolescents. Cochrane Database Syst Rev 2013;(7):CD002279.
15. Gao SS, Zhang S, Mei ML, et al. Caries remineralisation and arresting effect in children by professionally applied fluoride treatment: a systematic review. BMC Oral Health 2016;16:12.
16. Polyzos NP, Polyzos IP, Mauri D, et al. Effect of periodontal disease treatment during pregnancy on preterm birth incidence: a metaanalysis of randomized trials. Am J Obstet Gynecol 2009;200(3):225–32.
17. Jeffcoat MK, Hauth JC, Geurs NC, et al. Periodontal disease and preterm birth: results of a pilot intervention study. J Periodontol 2003;74(8):1214–8.
18. Han YW. Oral health and adverse pregnancy outcomes: what's next? J Dent Res 2011;90(3):289–93.
19. Fogacci MF, Leão A, Vettore MV, et al. Periodontal treatment completed before the 35th week of pregnancy appeared to have a beneficial effect on birthweight and time of delivery. Letter to the editor. J Dent Res 2010;89(2):101 [author reply: 101–2].
20. Novak T, Radnai M, Gorzó I, et al. Prevention of preterm delivery with periodontal treatment. Fetal Diagn Ther 2009;25(2):230–3.
21. Radnai M, Pál A, Novák T, et al. Benefits of periodontal therapy when preterm birth threatens. J Dent Res 2009;88(3):280–4.
22. Newnham JP, Shub A, Jobe AH, et al. The effects of intra-amniotic injection of periodontopathic lipopolysaccharides in sheep. Am J Obstet Gynecol 2005;193(2):313–21.
23. Shub A, Wong C, Jennings B, et al. Maternal periodontal disease and perinatal mortality. Aust N Z J Obstet Gynaecol 2009;49(2):130–6.
24. Milgrom P, Riedy CA, Weinstein P, et al. Design of a community-based intergenerational oral health study: "Baby Smiles". BMC Oral Health 2013;13:38.
25. Hummel J, et al. Organized, evidence-based care: oral health integration. In: Safety net medical home initiative. Seattle (WA): Qualis Health; 2016. p. 115.
26. Kaiser Family Foundation Key Facts about the Uninsured Population. 2018.
27. National Association of Dental Plans. Dental benefits basics 2017. Available at: https://www.nadp.org/Dental_Benefits_Basics/Dental_BB_1.aspx. Accessed April 15, 2019.
28. Centers for Disease Control and Prevention, National Diabetes Statistics Report 2017; Estimates of Diabetes and Its Burden in the United States. 2017.
29. Nasseh K, Vujicic M, Glick M. The relationship between periodontal interventions and healthcare costs and utilization. evidence from an integrated dental, medical, and pharmacy commercial claims database. Health Econ 2017;26(4):519–27.
30. Tonetti MS, Van Dyke TE, working group 1 of the joint EFP/AAP workshop. Periodontitis and atherosclerotic cardiovascular disease: consensus report of the

Joint EFP/AAP Workshop on Periodontitis and Systemic Diseases. J Periodontol 2013;84(4 Suppl):S24–9.

31. Park SY, Kim SH, Kang SH, et al. Improved oral hygiene care attenuates the cardiovascular risk of oral health disease: a population-based study from Korea. Eur Heart J 2019;40(14):1138–45.

32. Hong C, Aung MM, Kanagasabai K, et al. The association between oral health status and respiratory pathogen colonization with pneumonia risk in institutionalized adults. Int J Dent Hyg 2018;16(2):e96–102.

33. Palmer SC, Ruospo M, Wong G, et al. Dental health and mortality in people with end-stage kidney disease treated with hemodialysis: a multinational cohort study. Am J Kidney Dis 2015;66(4):666–76.

34. Ruospo M, Palmer SC, Craig JC, et al. Prevalence and severity of oral disease in adults with chronic kidney disease: a systematic review of observational studies. Nephrol Dial Transplant 2014;29(2):364–75.

35. Lee HJ, Choi EK, Park JB, et al. Tooth loss predicts myocardial infarction, heart failure, stroke, and death. J Dent Res 2019;98(2):164–70.

36. Brownlee B. Oral health integration in the patient-centered medical home (PCMH) environment: case studies from community health centers. Available at: https://www.dentaquestfoundation.org/sites/default/files/resources/Oral%20 Health%20Integration%20in%20the%20Patient-Centered%20Medical%20Home %2C%202012.pdf. Accessed April 15, 2019.

37. National Academy for State Health Policy. Case study: bridging medical and dental care at Marshfield Clinic and the Family Health Center. Available at: https://nashp. org/case-study-bridging-medical-dental-care-marshfield-clinic-family-health-center/. Accessed April 15, 2019.

38. Wall T, Nasseh K. Dental-related emergency department visits on the increase in the United States. May 2013. Available at: http://www.ada.org/media/ADA/Science% 20and%20Research/HPI/Files/HPIBrief_0513_1.ashx. Accessed November 26, 2013.

39. Olsen I, Singhrao SK, Osmundsen H. Periodontitis, pathogenesis and progression: miRNA-mediated cellular responses to *Porphyromonas gingivalis*. J Oral Microbiol 2017;9(1):1333396.

40. Pritchard AB, Crean S, Olsen I, et al. Periodontitis, microbiomes and their role in Alzheimer's disease. Front Aging Neurosci 2017;9:336.

41. Paganini-Hill A, White SC, Atchison KA. Dentition, dental health habits, and dementia: the Leisure World Cohort Study. J Am Geriatr Soc 2012;60(8):1556–63.

42. Ide M, Harris M, Stevens A, et al. Periodontitis and cognitive decline in Alzheimer's disease. PLoS One 2016;11(3):e0151081.

43. Kobayashi N, Soga Y, Maekawa K, et al. Prevalence of oral health-related conditions that could trigger accidents for patients with moderate-to-severe dementia. Gerodontology 2017;34(1):129–34.

44. Kobayashi T, Kubota M, Takahashi T, et al. Effects of tooth loss on brain structure: a voxel-based morphometry study. J Prosthodont Res 2018;62(3):337–41.

45. Braun PA, Cusick A. Collaboration between medical providers and dental hygienists in pediatric health care. J Evid Based Dent Pract 2016;16(Suppl):59–67.

46. Braun PA, Kahl S, Ellison MC, et al. Feasibility of colocating dental hygienists into medical practices. J Public Health Dent 2013;73(3):187–94.

47. Fisher-Owens SA. The primary teeth program: winner of the APA health care delivery award acceptance. Denver (CO): American Pediatric Association; 2011.

48. Ferullo A, Silk H, Savageau J. Teaching oral health in U.S. medical schools: results of a national survey. Acad Med 2011;86(2):226–30.

Caries Management Decision-Making
Diagnosis and Synthesis

Sandra Guzmán-Armstrong, DDS, MS[a],*,
David C. Johnsen, DDS, MS[b]

KEYWORDS

- Critical thinking • Decision-making • Caries • Management

KEY POINTS

- Offer a critical thinking skill set in decision-making and synthesis for caries diagnosis, and risk-adjusted and personalized management based on emulating the intended activity of the expert.
- Offer patient/case scenarios for application of the critical thinking skill set.
- Compare and contrast the result of applying an algorithm and expert thought process approach to patient analyses.
- Offer characteristics of the person making decisions and synthesizing information.
- For patients with complex health and social histories, include perspectives from other health care team members.

INTRODUCTION

The science of cariology continues to build as the science of caries management continues to build.[1–12] For the practitioner, 2 perspectives will determine success in managing caries: (1) an understanding of factors contributing to caries development and progression for the individual and (2) an understanding that these factors contribute to the presence and/or progression of the caries lesion as a manifestation of disease. For the educator, the challenge will be to translate the science into learning outcomes from which we can guide learning and assess performance at a level that will be accepted and implemented by peers. The challenge will be to translate the science and apply it to each patient to offer a comprehensive and personalized health-promoting and tooth-preserving strategy.[13]

Disclosure Statement: The authors have nothing to disclose.
[a] Department of Operative Dentistry, University of Iowa College of Dentistry and Dental Clinics, S-246 DSB, Iowa City, IA 52242-1001, USA; [b] Department of Pediatric Dentistry, University of Iowa College of Dentistry and Dental Clinics, Office of the Dean, N305 DSB, Iowa City, IA 52242-1010, USA
* Corresponding author.
E-mail address: sandra-guzman-armstrong@uiowa.edu

Dent Clin N Am 63 (2019) 679–693
https://doi.org/10.1016/j.cden.2019.06.007
dental.theclinics.com

Decision-making synthesizes and analyzes the main information gathered from the first 2 elements at the patient level (patients' caries risk assessment) and the lesion level (caries lesion classification and staging) resulting in a likelihood matrix that can guide the professional to assess whether new lesions will develop or existing lesions will progress over time (**Box 1, Figs. 1–3**), after which the practitioner can critically translate this information and produce a comprehensive and personalized caries management plan.

The purposes of this article are to: (1) offer a critical thinking skill set for caries risk assessment based on emulating the intended activity of the expert[14–16]—this approach follows an evolving critical thinking model in dentistry[17]; (2) offer patient/case scenarios for application of the critical thinking skill set; (3) compare and contrast the results of applying an algorithm and expert thought process approach to patient analyses; and (4) for patients with complex health and social histories, include perspectives from other health care team members. An assumption is made that persons with high caries levels have compounding health and social contributors.[18]

Box 1
Critical thinking applied to personalized risk-based caries management plan

- Gather basic data
  - Patient risk factors and history
  - Caries lesion classification: stage and activity
  - For patients with health and social complexities, incorporate interprofessional perspectives:
    - Prioritize the health conditions
    - Which of the patient's problems are drug related?
    - What is the patient's capacity to subscribe to recommended treatments?
    - Which of the patient's problems are nutrition related?
    - What are barriers to care?
    - Which of the patient's problems directly affect general health?

- Ask which data are important for the patient's health and why. Use evidence and rationale

- Ask what happens if we do nothing (ie, whether caries disease will progress or not)

- Determine the risk status based on disease progression/stage and which factors were likely causative:
  - Low-disease/low-risk factors: Low likelihood
  - Low-disease/high-risk factors: Moderate likelihood
  - High-disease/high-risk factors: High likelihood

- Ask what are alternatives with evidence and rationale to personalize a comprehensive caries risk-based management plan:
  - The patient's risk status (low, moderate, high) according to factors
  - Tooth-preserving management of caries lesions according to stage, activity, and likelihood of progression

- What is the specific recommendation and why: patient preference, evidence, and rationale?
  - Related to patient's risk factors
  - Related to caries lesion management (ie, prevention, nonrestorative care, tooth-preserving restorative care)

- What is the prognosis for the recommended treatment?

- What are your biases?

- Communications plan

- Self-assess: what was done well, what could be done better, and compare with peer assessment

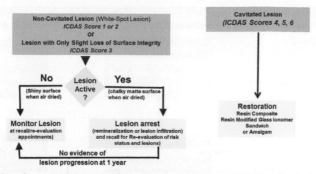

Fig. 1. Algorithm for management of noncavitated and cavitated caries lesions of smooth surfaces in permanent teeth. (*Courtesy of* the Department of Comprehensive Dentistry, University of Texas Health Science Center at San Antonio, San Antonio, TX; with permission.)

Critical thinking concepts are applied when providing rationale and synthesizing to solve a problem, because health care calls for inquiry and finding alternative explanations. The current literature is scant on the effective use of critical thinking skill sets in patient assessment and treatment planning. One promising approach builds on critical thinking concepts from the Education literature to emulate the intended activity of the expert.[19–22] These concepts have been used to design critical thinking skill sets in treatment planning, literature critique, and evidence-based dentistry,[23–25] as well as caries risk assessment.[16] The referenced caries risk assessment exercise successfully emulated the thought process of the expert in succinct enough fashion to be used by a novice in a clinical setting. One modification is to build in the dimension of time by including the state of disease progression. The risk assessment paradigm of "high," "moderate," and "low" alone does not offer the perspective of time. Because all patients are either progressing or reversing their health state, and none are static throughout their lifetime, this is an opportunity to include disease progression in the risk assessment, as has been done for the geriatric population.[26]

A Critical Thinking Skill Set Synthesizing Caries Lesion Diagnosis, and Caries Risk Assessment as a Precursor to Developing a Comprehensive Personalized Plan

Designing a critical thinking thought process for risk-based caries management depends on: (1) basic knowledge of caries pathology; (2) combining the concepts of

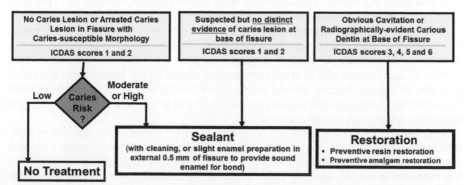

Fig. 2. Algorithm for management of caries lesions in occlusal surfaces of permanent teeth. (*Courtesy of* the Department of Comprehensive Dentistry, University of Texas Health Science Center at San Antonio, San Antonio, TX; with permission.)

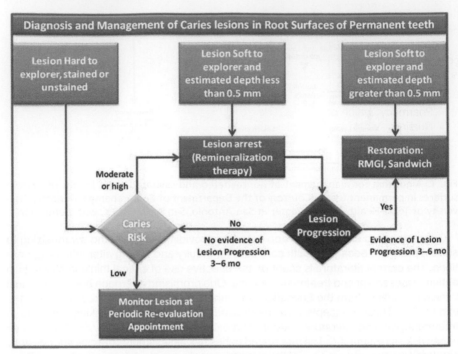

Fig. 3. Algorithm for management of root caries lesions in permanent teeth. RC, Resin composite restoration; RMGI, Resin modified glass ionomer; Sandwich, RMGI at gingival (Dentin) margin, RC on occlusal (Enamel). (*Courtesy of* the Department of Comprehensive Dentistry, University of Texas Health Science Center at San Antonio, San Antonio, TX; with permission.)

caries risk-based management plan with concepts in the Education literature on critical thinking; (3) direct emulation of the thought process of the expert; (4) viewing caries as a disease of the individual and viewing the caries lesion as a manifestation of the disease (tooth level), an approach that has been used for primary teeth[27-30]; and (5) for patients with complex health and social histories, inclusion of perspectives from other health care team members.

Although the act of conducting caries risk assessment by an experienced clinician can take place in a matter of seconds in a busy dental practice, novices learn this process by following specific steps practiced across the years of dental school that blend knowledge and critical thinking across disciplines. The final exercise demonstrating competence in performing individualized caries risk assessment is based on a solid foundation of knowledge, clinical exposure to patients, and case scenarios. First comes a basic understanding of the pathology of dental caries. Next comes an understanding of key risk factors, as well as classification of the activity and stage of each caries lesion.[31] Although it is beyond the scope of this article to offer an in-depth presentation, a summary is offered here.

After understanding the pathology and risk factors for dental caries, the use of algorithms (see **Figs. 1–3**) offers a powerful approach in preparation for following a thought process approach to caries lesion management. This process stipulates the dentist as the responsible person deciding upon the patient's condition and offering alternative intervention, with the patient making the final decision.

Because many patients have complexities in their health and social lives, a case is made for the dentist to incorporate the thought processes of fellow health team members in planning care. A compelling reason is that people with increased states of health risk and social risk are also at greater risk for caries.

The questions listed are derived from experts on the health care team but can be considered as "commonsense" questions. Identification of the health care provider is thus removed in **Box 1** on caries risk.

- Primary care: prioritize the health conditions
- Pharmacy: which of the patient's problems are drug related?
- Nursing: what is the patient's capacity to subscribe to recommended treatments?
- Nutrition: which of the patient's problems are nutrition related?
- Social work: what are barriers to care?
- Dentistry: which of the patient's problems directly affect general health?

The expert may not be able to articulate the thought process they are going through as situations arise.[32,33] A key for the novice or advanced beginner is to capture the thought process of the expert in succinct enough fashion for use in a clinical situation. A key concept in this progression is separation of learning the science of caries risk assessment from the critical thinking process of the accomplished clinician. Other critical thinking skill sets have been reported for dentistry.[17,22]

THE THOUGHT PROCESSES FOR ASSESSING CARIES DISEASE OF THE INDIVIDUAL AND ITS MANIFESTATION AT A TOOTH LEVEL ARE COMPLEMENTARY
The Algorithm-Based Thought Process in Assessing Caries Diagnosis and Treatment at a Tooth Level

Powerful algorithms are available in assessing caries for the tooth.[31] Success in arriving at a decision on treatment rests on a sound understanding of the pathology of caries and the factors contributing to caries. The algorithm leads to a treatment more than a set of alternatives for each individualized patient. The responsibility of executing the treatment rests with the clinician. For situations with the tooth as the isolated variable, the approach holds great promise.

The Thought Process for Assessing Caries Disease at a Patient Level as a Disease of the Individual and as a Manifestation of the Disease at a Tooth Level

The thought process for assessing caries for the person involves compounding variables that may lead more to alternatives than a "correct" treatment plan and subsequent procedures. A basic difference is in the nature of the questions asked, with greater demand on the judgment of the clinician. For example, "Which data are important?" is a different kind of question than "How deep is the lesion?" The same is true for "What happens if we do nothing?" Assessing risk without time can depict caries as static. Risk plus time helps to depict caries as dynamic.

Because all activity starts with articulating the thought process/skill set, the following are steps in the thought process of the expert in synthesizing an individual-based (rather than a tooth-based) personalized caries risk-based management plan (see **Box 1**). This is based on literature regarding characteristics of learning effectiveness or improvement. The process is designed to lead to alternatives before reaching a final recommendation for intervention.[14]

Key questions can quickly identify whether the practitioner understands the scope of the patient's condition. After gathering basic data, the first question of the expert should be, "Which data are important for the patient's health and why?" This question quickly focuses in on the practitioner's grasp of the larger context of the patient/case. In a similar vein, a next question may be, "What happens if I/we do nothing for some period of time (6 months or 5 years)?" This question also quickly focuses on the practitioner's grasp of the dynamic of the patient/case. The question leads to a prognosis with no treatment.

A next step is to determine the risk level and likelihood of new caries lesions and/or progression. Referencing risk to disease progression depicts the patient's situation and caries lesion itself as dynamic rather than static. For example, use of "high," "moderate," or "low" can depict a static situation. The risk orientation toward disease progression adds a time dynamic: low risk/low disease (low likelihood), high risk/low disease (moderate likelihood), high risk/rapidly progressing disease (high likelihood), extensive destruction/which factors contributed?

Once the risk is established, a next question is what are the alternatives, and what is the evidence and rationale for each? This focuses the clinician on synthesizing alternatives that target the patient's most relevant risk factors, the alternative tooth-preserving treatment options according the stage and activity of each lesion, the likelihood of progression, and creativity in developing alternatives. The habit of looking for alternatives rather than a "right" answer is consistent with the general occurrence in health care of alternatives more than "right" answers. Thus, different kinds of thinking are brought to bear in the process. Although algorithms are valuable, the dentist remains responsible for decisions.

Next is the decision to choose one alternative, calling on the patient's preference as well as the evidence and rationale. A next step is to assess one's biases. We all have them and many are healthy, yet it is essential to consider our biases.[34] Next is the communications plan with the patient, based on evidence and rationale. It is beyond the scope of this article to offer fundamentals of communication. Finally, self-assessment closes the loop on the process. Since self-assessment will be a key activity for success in practice, it is included in this and other thought processes.

Concepts in Critical Thinking Used to Design the Skill Set

Concepts underlie previously reported critical thinking skill sets for treatment planning, search and critique of the literature, and evidence-based dentistry, in addition to caries risk.[16,17,23–26] The following is a summary of the concepts underlying the aforementioned caries risk-based management skill set.

- Provide multiple (not endless) situations calling for critical thinking—the more situations, the more likely one is to adapt to new ones.
- Emulate the intended thinking as directly as possible.[14,19–22,35,36]
- Gain agreement of experts on content, application, and assessment.[21,22,37–39]
- Use the same instrument to guide learning and assess (or self-assess) performance.[40]
- Consider alternatives, biases (toward own abilities, patient conditions, and so forth), and self-assessment.[27]

PATIENT/CASE SCENARIOS

The use of patient/case scenarios can help to demonstrate the difference and complementary roles in assessing stage and progression for the tooth as well as assessing caries risk factors for the individual. A side-by-side comparison of the algorithm shown previously and the thought process/skill set of the expert show the key differences. The following 3 patients/cases demonstrate the application of the caries management thought process at a patient level and at a tooth level.

Patient/Case 1

- A 25-year-old who works night shifts in a convenience store selling gasoline, snack foods, and sweetened pop. Free beverage consumption is available for workers.
- The patient's medical history includes depression and anxiety. Antidepressant and antianxiety medications have been used for several years.
- The patient fails on the first appointment for an examination, keeps the second appointment, and fails the third appointment.
- The patient is slightly overweight but otherwise healthy. The patient has extensive tooth destruction from the caries process.

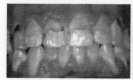 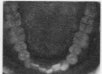 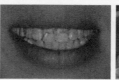 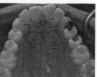

Front View   Lower Arch   Smile   Upper Arch

---

1. The thought process for assessing caries disease at a patient level

- Gather basic data

  - Patient risk factors and history. *High frequency and accessibility of sugar beverage and snacks, inconsistent oral hygiene because of work schedule, no history of restorative care and/or preventive care, medication-induced dry mouth, low socioeconomic status, thick plaque accumulation, low compliance*

  - Caries lesion classification: stage and activity. *Caries experience: initial, moderate, and extensive active caries lesions*

  - Health perspectives. *Nutrition: which of the patient's problems are diet related? Nursing: what is the patient's capacity to subscribe to recommended treatment? Social work: what are the barriers to care?*

- Ask which data are important for the patient's health and why. Use evidence and rationale. *Active caries lesions, lack of adequate fluoride exposure, high frequency and consumption of high-sugar beverages, irregular dental care, low socioeconomic status, low compliance, dry mouth, questionable ability and time to adhere to recommended interventions*

- Ask what happens if we do nothing (ie, will caries disease progress or not). *Caries disease will continue progressing, initial lesions will progress to moderate/extensive and eventually to possible dental sepsis. Sound tooth structure will develop new initial lesions*

- Determine the risk status based on disease progression/stage and which factors were likely causative.

  - *High-risk/rapidly progressing disease: high likelihood due to dry mouth, diet, lack of oral hygiene, lack of dental care*

- Ask what are alternatives with evidence and rationale to personalize a comprehensive caries risk-based management plan.

  - The patient's risk status (low, moderate, high) according to factors: *high risk*

  - Tooth-preserving management of caries lesions according to stage, activity, and likelihood of progression. *Placement pit and fissure sealants in all occlusal surfaces that have initial active lesions or susceptive pit and fissures, tooth brushing 2 times/day with high-fluoride prescription toothpaste, general behavior modification in oral hygiene, motivational engagement for dietary intake intervention and modification (reduce sugar amount and frequency), maintain dental visits at risk-based intervals, fluoride varnish application on active lesions 3 to 4 times a year. Tooth-preserving restorative care to moderate and extensive caries lesions. Altering medication-induced hyposalivation*

- What is the specific recommendation and why: patient preference, evidence, and rationale?
  - Related to patient's risk factors:
    - *Diet: motivational engagement for dietary intake intervention and modification, reducing amount and frequency of sugar beverages and providing alternatives such as water and sugar-free beverages with meals*
    - *Oral hygiene: professional cleaning, general behavior modification in oral hygiene, maintaining dental visits at risk-based intervals*
    - *Dry mouth: explore possibilities to modify medication-induced hyposalivation*
  - Related to caries lesion management (ie, prevention, nonrestorative care, tooth-preserving restorative care):
    - *Preventive care for sound tooth structure: preventive sealants, fluoride varnish application and tooth brushing 2 times/day with high-fluoride prescription toothpaste to prevent new lesions*
    - *Nonrestorative care for initial active caries lesions treatment: therapeutic sealants, fluoride varnish application, and tooth brushing 2 times/day with high-fluoride prescription toothpaste*
    - *Tooth-preserving restorative care for moderate and extensive caries lesions*
  - Prognosis with recommended intervention: *Moderate to poor given the social barriers and history of compliance*
- What are your biases? *Patient compliance, further rapid deterioration, patient may continue with inadequate diet and oral hygiene because of job schedule and availability of sugared beverages*
- Communications plan. *Discussion with patient of challenges at work having available sugar beverages for free and the need to compensate for dry mouth symptoms. Give alternatives to drink more ice-cold water and motivate the patient to modify diet and improve oral hygiene as well as exposure to high-fluoride toothpaste. Advise to complete recommended preventive, nonrestorative care and tooth-preserving restorative care treatment. Discuss the importance of applying fluoride varnish and maintaining dental visits at risk-based intervals. Recommend to discuss with physician alternatives to use noninduced hyposalivation medications*
- Self-assess: what was done well, what could be done better, and compare with peer assessment

2. The thought process for assessing caries disease at a tooth level (see **Figs. 1** and **2**)
   - Caries lesion classification
     - *Noncavitated lesion (white spot lesion), ICDAS (International Caries Detection and Assessment System) score 1 or 2*
     - *Suspected but not distinct evidence of caries lesion at base of fissure*
     - *Obvious cavitation, carious dentin at base of the fissure*
   - Caries risk: *high*
   - Lesion activity: *active*

- Treatment option for noncavitated lesions:
  - *Remineralization therapy or resin infiltration and recall for re-evaluation of risk status and lesions*
  - *If no evidence of lesion progression at 1 year, monitor lesion at recall appointments*
- Suspected but not distinct evidence of caries lesion at base of fissure:
  - *sealant*
- Treatment option for obvious cavitation:
  - *Preventive resin restoration*
  - *Preventive amalgam restoration*

A comparison of the 2 approaches ("algorithm" approach and the "expert thought process" approach) may be instructional to show how they complement each other. The advantage of the algorithm approach is a more focused treatment of the individual tooth. The advantage of deriving the thought process of the expert combines the risk of the individual tooth based on the pathologic state of the tooth and the risk of the individual.

Patient/Case 2

- A 23-year-old who has been a patient since childhood with low history of caries lesions and restorative care, few occlusal restorations and sealants before entering college, and no regular dental care after college.
- The patient is graduating from college and will be entering the Peace Corps with limited access to dental care for the next 3 years.
- During college the diet and oral hygiene slipped, and several initial caries lesions are noted.

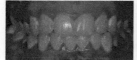 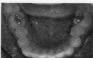 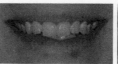 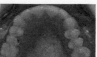

Front View   Lower Arch   Smile   Upper Arch

1. The thought process for assessing caries disease at a patient level
   - Gather basic data
     - Patient risk factors and history. *Changes in lifestyle (college) diet and oral hygiene deteriorating over time, thick plaque accumulation, history of few caries lesions and restorations, no regular dental care during college years*
     - Caries lesion classification: stage and activity. *Rampant initial active caries lesions*
     - Perspectives: Barriers to care? *Distance,* and Capacity to subscribe to treatment recommendations? *Limited with new lifestyle in the Peace Corps, diet uncertainties*
   - Ask which data are important for the patient's health and why. Use evidence and rationale. *History of caries disease, lack of adequate fluoride exposure, high-frequency and high-carbohydrate diet, irregular dental care, geographic separation from care for prolonged periods*

- Ask what happens if we do nothing (ie, will caries disease progress or not). *Caries disease will progress to moderate and eventually extensive stages. Patient will not have easy access to dental care in the near future*
- Determine the risk status based on disease progression/stage and which factors were likely causative.
  - *High-risk/rapidly progressing disease: High likelihood for progression because of diet, irregular dental care, low compliance, and poor oral hygiene*
- Ask what are alternatives with evidence and rationale to personalize a comprehensive caries risk-based management plan.
  - The patient's risk status (low, moderate, high) according to factors: *high risk*
  - Tooth-preserving management of caries lesions according to stage, activity, and likelihood of progression: *placement of pit and fissure sealants in all occlusal surfaces, tooth brushing 2 times/day with high-fluoride prescription toothpaste, general behavior modification in oral hygiene, motivational engagement for dietary intake intervention and modification, maintain dental visits at risk-based intervals, fluoride varnish application on active lesions 3 to 4 times a year*
- What is the specific recommendation and why: patient preference, evidence, and rationale
  - Related to patients' risk factors:
    - *Diet: motivational engagement for dietary intake intervention and modification*
    - *Oral hygiene: professional cleaning, general behavior modification in oral hygiene*
    - *History of few caries lesion and restorations: maintain dental visits to evaluate and maintain existing restorations*
    - *No regular dental care during college years: maintain dental visits at risk-based intervals*
  - Related to caries lesion management (ie, prevention, nonrestorative care, tooth-preserving restorative care)
    - *Preventive care: for sound tooth structure: preventive sealants, fluoride varnish application, and tooth brushing 2 times/day with high-fluoride prescription toothpaste to prevent new lesions*
    - *Nonrestorative care: for initial active caries lesions treatment: therapeutic sealants, fluoride varnish application, and tooth brushing 2 times/day with high-fluoride prescription toothpaste*
  - Prognosis for recommended treatment: *fair while in the Peace Corps and optimistic upon returning home*
- What are your biases? *Patient compliance and further rapid deterioration*
- Communications plan. *Discussion with patient of challenges in the near future to continue with consistent dental care and fluoride varnish application after going to Peace Corps for 3 years, reinforce the importance to modify diet and improve oral hygiene as well as access to high-fluoride toothpaste and the possibility to carry more tubes of prescription toothpaste. Advise to complete recommended preventive and nonrestorative care treatment as soon as possible before patient leaves to join Peace Corps*
- Self-assess: what was done well, what could be done better, and compare with peer assessment

2. The thought process in assessing caries diagnosis at a tooth level (see **Fig. 1**)
   - Caries lesion classification: *noncavitated lesion (white spot lesion), ICDAS score 1 or 2*
   - Lesion activity: *active*

- Treatment option:
  - *Remineralization therapy or resin infiltration and recall for re-evaluation of risk status and lesions*
  - *If no evidence of lesion progression at 1 year, monitor lesion at recall appointments*

Patient/Case 3

- A long-time patient now 80 years old with beginning dementia and Parkinson disease as well as indication of dry mouth caused by multiple medications
- At age 55 the patient had extensive fixed prosthodontics
- Early signs of active initial root surface caries, and initial caries lesions adjacent to restorations
- Oral hygiene quality and frequency has deteriorated over time
- The family is aware of the possibility of entering a nursing home in the next few years

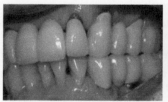 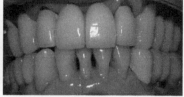

    Front View   Front View

1. The thought process for assessing caries disease at a patient level

- Gather basic data
  - Patient risk factors and history. *Exposed root surfaces, dry mouth caused by medications, inadequate oral hygiene, deficient exposure to topical fluoride, systematic compromised patient (changes in lifestyle), restorations; deficient restoration, marginal adaptation*
  - Caries lesion classification: stage and activity. *Initial active caries lesions*
  - Perspectives. *Pharmacy: multiple medications and dry mouth; Nursing: capacity to subscribe to treatments; Social work: barriers to care*
  - Ask which data are important for the patient's health and why. Use evidence and rationale. *Systematic compromised patient, lifestyle changes, poor oral hygiene and fluoride exposure, dry mouth, limited ability to subscribe to treatment, difficulty accessing appointments, multiple medications and dry mouth*
- Ask what happens if we do nothing (ie, will caries disease progress or not). *Caries disease will progress from initial to extensive caries disease*
- Determine the risk status based on disease progression/stage and which factors were likely causative.
  - *High-risk/rapidly progressive disease: dry mouth, poor oral hygiene/fluoride exposure, heavily restored with multiple restorations with deficient marginal adaptation*

- Ask what are alternatives with evidence and rationale to personalize a comprehensive caries risk-based management plan.
  - The patient's risk status (low, moderate, high) according to factors: *high risk owing to initial disease and significant risk factors such as lifestyle changes caused by Parkinson disease, dementia, dry mouth, poor oral hygiene, and fluoride exposure and restorations*
  - Tooth-preserving management of caries lesions according to stage, activity, and likelihood of progression: *Tooth brushing 2 times/day with high-fluoride prescription toothpaste, improve oral hygiene and fluoride exposure (electric toothbrush), chlorhexidine varnish, saliva stimulation, if possible altering dry mouth–induced medication, motivational engagement to educate the patient and patient's family about changes and to be aware of high-sugar, high-frequency dietary intake, maintain dental visits at risk-based intervals, fluoride varnish application*
- What is the specific recommendation and why: patient preference, evidence, and rationale
  - Related to patients' risk factors:
    - *Fluoride: increase exposure and concentration*
    - *Oral hygiene: professional cleaning, improve oral hygiene*
    - *Dry mouth: if possible altering dry mouth–induced medication*
    - *Maintain dental visits at risk-based intervals*
  - Related to caries lesion management (ie, prevention, nonrestorative care, tooth-preserving restorative care):
    - *Preventive care: for sound tooth structure: fluoride varnish application 2 times per year*
    - *Nonrestorative care: root initial lesions treatment with chlorhexidine varnish and/or fluoride varnish, silver diamine fluoride (SDF)*
  - Prognosis: *moderate with good family and institutional support; poor with limited family and social support*
- What are your biases? *Poor patient compliance with inability to comply without help*
- Communications plan. *Discussion with patient and patient's family about challenges while undergoing medical treatment and future systemic conditions as well as lifestyle changes in nursing home. Educate patient of possible changes and to continue with risk-based dental care, fluoride, and chlorhexidine varnish application. Reinforce the importance of low-sugar, low-frequency diet and improve oral hygiene and increase dental visits*
- Self-assess: what was done well, what could be done better, and compare with peer assessment

2. The thought process in assessing caries diagnosis at a tooth level (see **Fig. 3**)
  - Caries lesion classification:
    - *Lesion difficult to explore; stained and unstained*
  - Caries risk: *high*
  - Lesion activity: *active*
  - Treatment option for noncavitated lesions:
    - *Remineralization therapy or SDF and recall for re-evaluation of risk status and lesions*
    - *If no evidence of lesion progression at 3 to 6 months, monitor lesion at recall appointments*
    - *If lesion progression, initiate restorative care (resin composite, resin-modified glass ionomers, or sandwich)*

A comparison of the 2 approaches in caries risk is instructional to enhance complementary application. The algorithm approach allows management of the individual tooth, but is limited in factoring of general health problems such as dementia, Parkinson disease, stroke, and dry mouth. These health problems need the perspectives of pharmacy, nutrition, and social work to be systematically included in a thought process used by the expert. This thought process leads to alternatives before selecting a final intervention. Patients like the one described here involve compromises, so there may not be a "correct" answer agreeable to a spectrum of clinicians. A shortcoming of the algorithm approach is evident in situations where a compromise will be likely.

SUMMARY

The use of patient/case scenarios can help to demonstrate the difference and complementary roles in assessing stage and progression for the tooth as well as assessing caries risk factors for the individual. Several key points summarize this article, the first of which is the importance of viewing caries as a disease at the individual level and the manifestation of disease at the tooth level. This rests on a sound knowledge of the pathology and factors contributing to caries. It also rests on a sense of the relative weight of factors contributing to the rapidity of caries progression for the individual patient. For assessment of the lesion as manifestation of the disease, algorithms leading to a definitive diagnosis and treatment plan can be useful to guide clinical success. For caries risk assessment of the individual, there should be a progression to master a thought process synthesizing contributing factors, leading to alternatives for the patient to choose a specific intervention. The 2 approaches are viewed as complementary.

ACKNOWLEDGMENTS

The authors would like to acknowledge Dr. Leo Marchini for his contribution by reviewing the content and providing feedback.

REFERENCES

1. Teich ST, Demko C, Al-Rawa W, et al. Assessment of implementation of a CAMBRA-based program in a dental school environment. J Dent Educ 2013; 77(4):438–47.
2. Ismail AI, Tellez M, Pitts NB, et al. Caries management pathways preserve dental tissues and promote oral health. Community Dent Oral Epidemiol 2013;41: e12–40.
3. Pitts NB, Ekstrand KR, ICDAS Foundation. International Caries Detection and Assessment System (ICDAS) and its International Caries Classification and Management System (ICCMS)—methods for staging of the caries process and enabling dentists to manage caries. Community Dent Oral Epidemiol 2013;41: e41–52.
4. Jenson L, Budenz AW, Featherstone JD, et al. Clinical protocols for caries management by risk assessment. J Calif Dent Assoc 2007;35(10):714–23.
5. Featherstone JD, Domejean-Orliaguet S, Jenson L, et al. Caries risk assessment in practice for age 6 through adult. J Calif Dent Assoc 2007;35(10):703–7, 710–3.
6. Young DA, Featherstone JD, Roth JR, et al. Caries management by risk assessment: implementation guidelines. J Calif Dent Assoc 2007;35(11):799–805.
7. Powell LV. Caries prediction: a review of the literature. Community Dent Oral Epidemiol 1998;26:361–71.

692   Guzmán-Armstrong & Johnsen

8. Fontana M, Zero DT. Assessing patients' caries risk. J Am Dent Assoc 2006; 137(9):1231-9.

9. Marshall TA. Chairside diet assessment of caries risk. J Am Dent Assoc 2009; 140(6):670-4.

10. Meyer-Lueckel H, Paris S, Ekstrand K. Caries management: science and clinical practice. New York: Thieme Editions; 2013.

11. Shaffer JR, Wang X, Feingold E, et al. Genome-wide association scan for childhood caries implicates novel genes. J Dent Res 2011;90(12):1457-62.

12. Slayton RL, Urquhart O, Araujo MWB, et al. Evidence-based clinical practice guideline on nonrestorative treatments for carious lesions. J Am Dent Assoc 2018;149(10):837-49.

13. Fontana M, Pilcher L, Tampi MP, et al. J Am Dent Assoc 2018;149(11):935-7.

14. Johnsen DC, Lipp MJ, Finkelstein MW, et al. Guiding dental student learning and assessing performance in critical thinking with analysis of emerging strategies. J Dent Educ 2012;76(12):1548-58.

15. Johnsen DC. Critical thinking: focal point for a culture of inquiry. In: Boyle C, editor. Student learning: improving practice. Hauppauge (NY): Nova Science Publishing; 2013. p. 151-70.

16. Guzman-Armstrong S, Warren J, Cunningham-Ford M, et al. Concepts in critical thinking applied to caries risk assessment. J Dent Educ 2014;78(6):914-20.

17. Marshall TA, Marchini L, Cowen H, et al. Critical thinking theory to practice: using the expert's thought process as guide for learning and assessment. J Dent Educ 2017;81(9):978-85.

18. Johnsen DC, Pappas LR, Cannon D, et al. Social factors and diet diaries of caries-free and high-caries 2- to 7-year olds presenting for dental care in West Virginia. Pediatr Dent 1980;2(4):279-86.

19. Baron JB. Strategies for the development of effective performance exercises. Appl Meas Educ 1991;4(4):305-18.

20. Bauer BA. A study of the reliability and cost-effectiveness of three methods of assessment for writing ability. ERIC Document Reproduction Service; 1981. No. 216357. Available at: https://eric.ed.gov/?id=ED216357.

21. Clauser BE. Recurrent issues and recent advances in scoring performance assessments. Appl Psychol Meas 2000;24(4):310-24.

22. Lane S, Stone CA. Performance assessment. In: Brennan RL, editor. Educational measurement. 4th edition. Westport (CT): National Council on Measurement in Education, Praeger Publishers; 2006. p. 1-112.

23. Johnsen DC, Finkelstein MW, Marshall TA, et al. A model for critical thinking measurement of dental school performance. J Dent Educ 2009;73(2):177-83.

24. Straub-Morarend CL, Marshall TA, Holmes DC, et al. Informational resources utilized in clinical decision making: common practices in dentistry. J Dent Educ 2011;75(4):441-52.

25. Marshall TA, Straub-Morarend CL, Handoo N, et al. Integrating critical thinking and evidence-based dentistry across a four-year dental curriculum: a model for independent learning. J Dent Educ 2014;78(3):359-67.

26. Marchini L, Hartshorn JE, Cowen H, et al. Teaching tool for establishing risk of oral health deterioration in elderly patients: development, implementation, and evaluation at a US dental school. J Dent Educ 2017;81(11):1283-90.

27. Douglass JM, Tinanoff N, Tang JMW, et al. Dental caries patterns and oral health behaviors in Arizona infants and toddlers. Community Dent Oral Epidemiol 2001; 29:14-22.

28. Tsai AI, Chen C-Y, Li L-A, et al. Risk indicators for early childhood caries in Taiwan. Community Dent Oral Epidemiol 2006;34:437–45.
29. Johnsen DC, Bhat M, Kim MT, et al. Caries levels and patterns in head start children in fluoridated and non-fluoridated urban and non-urban sites in Ohio, USA. Community Dent Oral Epidemiol 1986;14:206–10.
30. Johnsen DC, Schubot D, Bhat M, et al. Caries pattern identification in the primary dentition: a comparison of clinician assignment and clinical analysis groupings. Pediatr Dent 1993;13:113–5.
31. Amaechi BT, van Amerongen JP, van Loveren C, et al. Caries management: diagnosis and treatment strategies. In: Hilton TJ, Ferracane JL, Broome JC, editors. Summitt's fundamentals of operative dentistry. 4th edition. New Malden (UK): Quintessence Publishing; 2013. p. 93–130.
32. Benner P. The Dreyfus model of skill acquisition applied to nursing. In: Benner P, editor. From novice to expert. Menlo Park (CA): Addison-Wesley; 2001. p. 13–38.
33. Leary KS, Marchini L, Hartshorn J, et al. An emulation model in critical thinking used to develop learning outcomes in inter professional practice. Clin Exp Dent Res 2019. https://doi.org/10.1002/cre2.195.
34. Kahneman D. Thinking fast and slow. New York: Farrar, Straus, and Giroux; 2011.
35. Baron J. Thinking and deciding. 4th edition. Cambridge (England): Cambridge University Press; 2008.
36. Messick S. The interplay of evidence and consequences in the validation of performance assessments. Educ Res 1994;23(2):13–23.
37. Frederiksen JR, Collins A. A systems approach to educational testing. Educ Res 1989;18(9):27–32.
38. Haertel EH, Linn RL. Comparability. In: Phillips GW, editor. Technical issues in large-scale performance assessment, NCES 96-802. Washington, DC: U.S. Department of Education; 1996. p. 59–78.
39. Marzano RJ, Pickering RJ, McTighe J. Assessing student outcomes: performance assessment using the dimensions of learning model. Alexandria (VA): Association for Su- pervision and Curriculum Development; 1993.
40. Kane M, Crooks T, Cohen A. Validating measures of performance. Educ Meas Issues Pract 1999;18(2):5–17.

Nonrestorative Management of Cavitated and Noncavitated Caries Lesions

Margherita Fontana, DDS, PhD

KEYWORDS

- Dental caries • Caries lesion • Noncavitated • Cavitated • Remineralization • Arrest
- Reversal

KEY POINTS

- To manage the caries disease process, a patient with active caries lesions needs a combination of strategies directed at the level of the individual to reduce the risk of caries and prevent future caries lesions and then additionally requires tooth-level strategies specifically targeted to manage existing caries lesions.
- Clinicians should consider thresholds for restorative and nonrestorative interventions for dental caries lesion management in the context of the patient, dentist, and existing evidence. Clinicians should strive to provide personalized or specific interventions with the highest levels of supporting evidence whenever possible.
- For cavitated lesions, evidence-based nonrestorative effective alternatives are limited, for example, silver diamine fluoride.
- For noncavitated lesions, effective strategies vary by tooth surfaces.
- Caries lesions treated nonrestoratively should be monitored over time, to assess the efficacy of interventions.

INTRODUCTION

Dental caries, a multifactorial disease process, results from a dysbiosis in the oral biofilm, stimulated by frequent exposure to fermentable carbohydrates, which over time results in demineralization of dental hard tissues.[1,2] Currently, caries management involves a conservative and preventive evidence-based philosophy, with person-centered risk-based disease management, early detection of caries lesions, and efforts to reverse and/or arrest caries lesions, with the aim to preserve tooth structure and maintain health.[2–4] To facilitate implementation of this philosophy, guidelines have been developed to aid in clinical decision making between restorative and nonrestorative interventions for caries lesions.[5] Guidelines also have been developed to identify what the best evidence-based strategies are for nonrestorative management

Department of Cariology, Restorative Sciences and Endodontics, University of Michigan School of Dentistry, 1011 North University, Room 2393, Ann Arbor, MI 48109, USA
E-mail address: mfontan@umich.edu

Dent Clin N Am 63 (2019) 695–703
https://doi.org/10.1016/j.cden.2019.06.001
0011-8532/19/© 2019 Elsevier Inc. All rights reserved.

of caries lesions of different severity in primary and permanent teeth and in different locations of the tooth structure.[6,7]

CARIES LESION CHARACTERISTICS THAT INFLUENCE TREATMENT DECISION MAKING

The accurate detection and assessment of existing caries lesions, and their monitoring over time, are essential steps in the diagnostic process leading to a clinical decision about how to best manage, in a person-centered manner, both the disease and the resulting caries lesions.[7,8]

If an active dental caries disease process develops in a tooth surface (ie, where acids derived from the metabolism of oral biofilms result in more demineralization than remineralization of tooth structure over a period of time), and this is allowed to continue unmanaged, over time the disease results in the development of detectable changes in the tooth structure, or caries lesions. In the beginning, these caries lesions are noncavitated (ie, macroscopically intact, sometimes referred to as white spot lesions) but eventually might progress to cavitation (ie, referred to as a cavity, where there is a break in the tooth surface, usually determined using visual or tactile means).[2,9,10] Because the activity of the caries disease process can vary over time (eg, the risk for dental caries can change as individuals, for example, change their oral hygiene or dietary habits), caries lesions also can go through stages of progression and arrest throughout the life time. This can happen naturally (through exposure to saliva, self-cleaning, and so forth) or can be aided with products and/or interventions (nonrestorative as well as restorative). In general, it is more difficult to arrest caries lesions once they are cavitated, unless they are restored, because oral biofilms are infecting dental tissues and thus are difficult to access for control. Furthermore, caries lesions can be located in different tissues (ie, enamel vs dentin) and surfaces (eg, occlusal, proximal, and root), which allows for different clinical access and may require different interventions.[2] Lesions also may be active or arrested, which also influences the need or not for intervention from a disease perspective.

A recent expert-based consensus report suggested that for best management, a caries lesion's cavitation, cleansability, and activity need to be considered. The report also provided recommendations for thresholds between restorative and nonrestorative interventions.[5] Thus, the following recommendations can help guide when use of nonrestorative strategies may be most appropriate[5,8]:

- Arrested caries lesions do not need to be treated from a caries disease perspective (either restoratively or nonrestoratively [**Fig. 1**]), except when the goal is to address issues associated with esthetics, function, or risk for pulpal death.
- Noncavitated active caries lesions should be treated using evidence-based nonrestorative products or interventions.
  - Some occlusal noncavitated lesions might extend radiographically deep into dentin. These lesions can be treated nonrestoratively (eg, using sealants), but it has been suggested that a trampoline effect (ie, in which the surface of the lesion may cavitate, because the body of the lesion is extensive and may undermine it) may result in the sealant failing, and thus treatment should be closely monitored.[5]
- Cavitated caries lesions (**Fig. 2**) generally are noncleansable and thus active; therefore, these lesions most commonly need to be restored. Selective removal of carious tissues[11] is guided by the depth of the lesion, pulpal health, and choice of dental material. Restoration of the existing cavity allows for oral biofilms to be relocated to the surface of the tooth and amenable to better control of the local

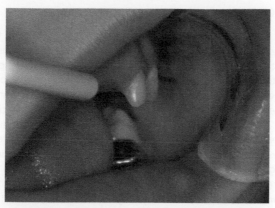

Fig. 1. Example of a noncavitated caries lesion in a mesial coronal surface of a primary incisor. Because the lesion is now cleansable and smooth, the lesion is considered arrested and not in need of caries intervention.

disease process. In addition, restoring the cavity allows for re-establishment of function and esthetics, which can be important patient-level outcomes.

- Some cavitated lesions that are not pulpally involved could be treated nonrestoratively (eg, with silver diamine fluoride [SDF]), either temporarily or permanently, if the primary goal is to arrest the caries disease process, with the understanding that function and esthetics remain compromised because of the loss of tooth structure. For some individuals, because of medical, social, behavioral, and/or financial factors, this compromise is the most appropriate person-centered approach to managing appropriate cavitated lesions.

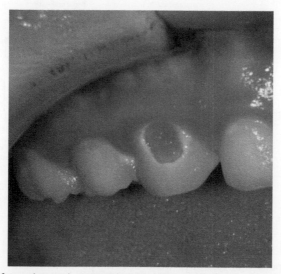

Fig. 2. Example of an advanced cavitated caries lesion with dentin clinically exposed in the facial coronal surface of a primary canine. Because dentin is soft on gentle probing, the lesion is considered active and in need of intervention.

NONRESTORATIVE CARIES LESION TREATMENT OPTIONS

Clinicians should consider options for nonrestorative interventions for dental caries lesion management in the context of the patient, dentist, and, whenever possible, the highest levels of supporting evidence. Clinical decision making must take into consideration patient caries risk, readiness for change, and likelihood of compliance with the proposed interventions.[2,9] Systematic reviews[12] and evidence-based practice guidelines for nonrestorative treatment options were published recently by the American Dental Association (ADA) (**Figs. 3** and **4**).[7] Although this article does not discuss risk assessment and caries prevention, it is imperative to remember that to manage the caries disease process, a patient with active caries lesions needs a combination of strategies directed at the level of the individual to reduce the risk of caries and prevent future caries lesions and then additionally requires tooth-level strategies (some of them nonrestorative), specifically targeted to manage existing caries lesions. Evidence-based nonrestorative treatment alternatives are discussed.

Fluoride

Beyond fluoride's important role in caries prevention for primary and permanent teeth at individual and community levels, and the fact that daily use of a fluoride-containing toothpaste is universally recommended to all dentate individuals for caries prevention, clinical evidence also supports the use of fluoride for caries lesion arrest and/or reversal.[2] Based on a 2018 ADA systematic review and subsequent evidence-based practice guidelines, the following fluoride products are recommended as effective for arresting and/or reversing caries lesions[7,12]:

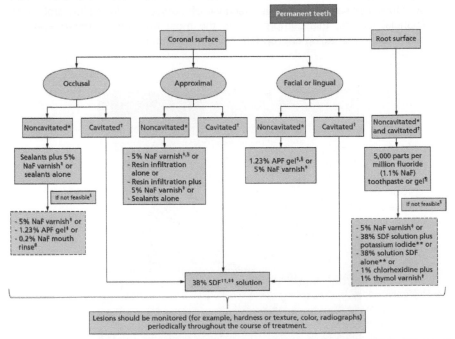

Fig. 3. Recommended nonrestorative treatments for permanent teeth. (*From* Slayton R, Urquhart O, Araujo MB. Evidence-based clinical practice guideline on nonrestorative treatments for caries lesions: A report from the American Dental Association. J Am Dent Assoc. 2018; 149(10):846; with permission.)

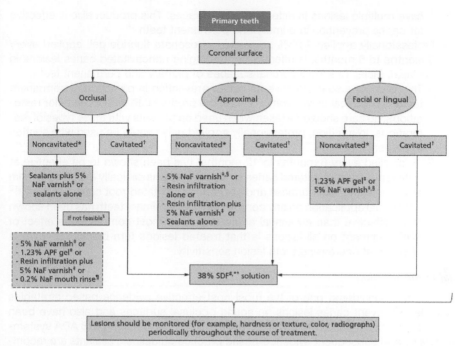

Fig. 4. Recommended nonrestorative treatments for primary teeth. (*From* Slayton R, Urquhart O, Araujo MB. Evidence-based clinical practice guideline on nonrestorative treatments for caries lesions: A report from the American Dental Association. J Am Dent Assoc. 2018; 149(10):845; with permission.)

- A 5000-ppm fluoride dentifrice or gel (1.1% sodium fluoride [NaF]), used at least once per day, is effective for root surface cavitated and noncavitated caries lesion control. Evidence from a network meta-analysis also suggests that of all available effective strategies to arrest caries lesions on root surfaces, a 5000-ppm fluoride dentifrice or gel is the most effective.[12]
  - These products require a prescription in the United States. The effectiveness of these high-fluoride products for root caries lesion arrest is not unexpected, because dentin tissues, compared with enamel, require higher levels of fluoride to obtain the same level of remineralization.[13] Furthermore, use of these products not only helps with managing root caries lesions but also helps prevent caries lesions in other tooth surfaces.[14]
- A 0.2% NaF mouth rinse, used once per week, is effective for controlling noncavitated lesions in the occlusal surfaces of primary and permanent teeth.
  - This product requires a prescription in the United States. Care must be taken to not use fluoride mouth rinses in young children until they can expectorate on demand. In addition, this product is effective at preventing caries experience.[15,16]
- Professionally applied 5% fluoride varnish (NaF), applied every 3 months to 6 months, is effective for managing noncavitated caries lesions in all coronal and root tooth surfaces of primary and permanent teeth. Also, a 5% NaF varnish is the most effective treatment alternative for arresting/reversing noncavitated lesions on coronal facial/lingual lesions of primary and permanent teeth.[12]
  - The fact that this product works on all tooth surfaces is particularly important for decisions on how to arrest/reverse caries lesions in at-risk patients who

have multiple lesions in different tooth surfaces. This product also is effective for caries prevention in primary and permanent teeth.[16]

- Professionally applied 1.23% acidulated phosphate fluoride gel, applied every 3 months to 6 months, is effective for managing noncavitated caries lesions in occlusal, facial, or lingual coronal surfaces of primary and permanent teeth.
  - This product also is effective for caries prevention in primary and permanent teeth.[17] A clinical consideration is that the product can etch tooth color restorations, so care should be taken when used on patients with these types of restorations. In addition, professionally applied gels should be used with suction to prevent ingestion.
- SDF, applied every 6 months to 12 months, has been shown to be effective at arresting advanced cavitated caries lesions (ie, lesions clinically exposing dentin) in all coronal and root surfaces and also on noncavitated root caries lesions.[7,12]
  - A biannual application on any coronal surface of primary teeth has been shown more effective than an annual application. The most common side effect of SDF treatment on all lesions is that treated lesions turn black. SDF also is effective at decreasing tooth lesion sensitivity.

Sealants/Infiltration

Sealants are considered one of the most cost-effective evidence-based strategies available to prevent caries lesions on sound occlusal surfaces and also have been advocated to arrest noncavitated caries lesions.[2,18,19] Based on a 2018 ADA systematic review and subsequent evidence-based practice guidelines, sealants are recommended as an effective treatment for arresting the following caries lesions[7,12]:

- Sealants are effective at arresting noncavitated lesions in occlusal and proximal coronal surfaces of primary and permanent teeth.
  - On occlusal surfaces, sealants can be used either alone or in combination with 5% NaF varnish (applied every 3–6 months). A recent systematic review concluded, however, that a combination of sealant plus 5% NaF varnish is the most effective strategy in arresting/reversing noncavitated occlusal lesions.[12]
  - Because a recent systematic review concluded that is it unclear which type of sealant material is more effective for caries control,[20] the decision of which material to choose should take into account the likelihood of loss of retention over time (ie, resin-based materials have significantly higher retention rates than glass ionomer [GI] materials) and the possibility of obtaining a dry field control during sealant placement (ie, GI materials are more hydrophilic).[20]
  - Limited data suggest that sealants also be may effective at arresting lesion progression when used on small cavitated or microcavitated lesions.[21] A recent systematic review and meta-analysis concluded, however, that when used on these type of lesions, current sealant materials require more repairs over time than minimally invasive restorations.[22]

Although sealants also are recommended to arrest noncavitated lesions in interproximal surfaces, these lesions normally are not accessible, and thus the procedure requires a second visit after tooth separation to be completed. Thus, infiltration of noncavitated lesions (ie, if not visible by direct observation, assessed based on radiographic depth as into enamel or outer third of dentin) has been developed as an alternative to be used in a single appointment. Based on a 2018 ADA systematic review and subsequent evidence-based practice guidelines, infiltration is recommended as an effective treatment for arresting the following caries lesions[7,12]:

- Using infiltration, whether alone or in combination with a 5% NaF varnish application every 3 months to 6 months, is effective at arresting interproximal coronal noncavitated caries lesions.
  - Because the infiltrant material currently is not radiopaque, the way to evaluate success of lesion arrest is by monitoring the radiographic lack of lesion progression over time.

Antimicrobials

Because dental caries results from a dysbiosis in the oral biofilm, restoring balance within that biofilm (through the use of antimicrobials, prebiotics, probiotics, and so forth) has been advocated.[23] Although chlorhexidine is one of the most commonly investigated antimicrobial strategies for caries control and prevention, current evidence suggests that chlorhexidine rinses (0.2% or 0.12%) are not effective at reducing dental caries.[24] Evidence, however, supports the use of 1% chlorhexidine varnish for the prevention of root caries lesions.[24] Based on a 2018 ADA systematic review and subsequent evidence-based practice guidelines, chlorhexidine is recommended as effective to arrest the following caries lesions[7,12]:

- Professional application of 1% chlorhexidine plus 1% thymol varnish, applied every 3 months to 6 months, is effective to arrest noncavitated or cavitated root caries lesions.

In addition, an alternative that has been suggested in the literature to enhance control of oral biofilms and arrest caries lesions is the so-called nonrestorative caries treatment approach. In this intervention, cavitated caries lesions that have limited cleansability, are opened up (with either hand instruments or a hand piece) to enhance cleansability, access of saliva, and decrease food retention. A recent randomized clinical trial in primary teeth concluded this treatment alternative was as effective as conventional restorative treatment in managing cavitated lesions in primary teeth.[25]

Calcium-based Strategies

A variety of products containing calcium in different forms (calcium attached to casein derivatives, calcium sodium phosphosilicate, and so forth) have been introduced to aid with caries lesion prevention and remineralization. The evidence supporting the clinical efficacy of these products is still either limited or inconsistent.[24] Based on a 2018 ADA systematic review and subsequent evidence-based practice guidelines, the following was recommended[7,12]:

- 10% casein phosphopeptide-amorphous calcium phosphate is not recommended as effective to arrest or reverse noncavitated carious lesions on coronal surfaces of primary and permanent teeth.
  - In particular, it was emphasized that this product should not be used as a substitute for fluoride products or if other fluoride interventions, sealants, or resin infiltration are accessible.

In addition, separate reports have concluded that promising clinical evidence suggests that the use of a prebiotic, such as arginine, to modulate dysbiotic dental biofilms, in combination with fluoride and calcium carbonate, has the ability to enhance the anticaries and remineralization effects of fluoride.[26] Yet all the existing clinical trials have been conducted to date by the manufacturer, and most are short term.[27] The product tested in these trials is currently not available in the United States.

SUMMARY

Although the existing evidence on arresting or reversing caries lesions on primary and permanent teeth and different tooth surfaces is more limited than the evidence for use of strategies to prevent development of new caries lesions, there are recent efforts to identify this literature and develop evidence-based practice guidelines. Clinicians should consider thresholds for restorative and nonrestorative interventions in the context of the patient, dentist, and existing evidence and should strive to provide interventions with the highest levels of supporting evidence whenever accessible. For cavitated lesions, nonrestorative alternatives are limited, with most trials focused on use of SDF. For noncavitated lesions, effective strategies in many cases vary by tooth surfaces. Tooth-level approaches need to be combined with strategies to manage the caries disease process at the individual level and prevent new caries lesions over time.

REFERENCES

1. Fontana M, Wolff M, Featherstone JBD. Introduction to ICNARA 3. Adv Dent Res 2018;29(1):3.
2. Fontana M, Gonzalez-Cabezas C. EBD caries risk assessment and disease management. Dent Clin North Am 2019;63:119–28.
3. Slayton RL, Fontana M, Young D, et al. Dental caries management in children and adults. In: Discussion Paper, National Academy of Medicine, Washington, DC 2016. Available at: https://nam.edu/wp-content/uploads/2016/09/Dental-Caries-Management-in-Children-and-Adults.pdf. Accessed May 6, 2018.
4. Fontana M, González-Cabezas C. Noninvasive caries risk-based management in private practice settings may lead to reduced caries experience over time. J Evid Based Dent Pract 2016;16(4):239–42.
5. Schewendicke F, Frenchen J, Bjørndal L, et al. Managing carious lesions: recommendations on carious tissue removal. Adv Dent Res 2016;28:58–67.
6. Ismail AI, Tellez M, Pitts NB, et al. Caries management pathways preserve dental tissues and promote oral health. Community Dent Oral Epidemiol 2013;41(1): e12–40.
7. Slayton R, Urquhart O, Araujo MB, et al. Evidence-based clinical practice guideline on nonrestorative treatments for caries lesions: a report from the American Dental Association. J Am Dent Assoc 2018;149(10):837–49.
8. Fontana M, Huysmans MC. Clinical decion-making in caries management: role of caries detection and diagnosis. In: Zandona A, Longbottom C, editors. Detection and assessment of dental caries – a clinical guide: Springer, in press.
9. Fontana M, Young D, Wolff M, et al. Defining dental caries for 2010 and beyond. Dent Clin North Am 2010;54:423–40.
10. Fontana M, Gonzalez-Cabezas C, Fitzgerald M. Cariology for the 21st century-current caries management concepts for dental practice. J Mich Dent Assoc 2013;95(4):32–40.
11. Innes N, Frenchen J, Bjørndal L, et al. Managing carious lesions: recommendations on terminology. Adv Dent Res 2016;28:49–57.
12. Urquhart O, Tampi MP, Pilcher L, et al. Nonrestorative treatments for caries: systematic review and network meta-analysis. J Dent Res 2018;1–13. https://doi.org/10.1177/0022034518800014.
13. ten Cate JM, Damen JJ, Buijs MJ. Inhibition of dentin demineralization by fluoride in vitro. Caries Res 1998;32(2):141–7.

14. Weyant RJ, Tracy SL, Anselmo TT, et al. Topical fluoride for caries prevention: executive summary of the updated clinical recommendations and supporting systematic review. J Am Dent Assoc 2013;144(11):1279–91.
15. Marinho VC, Chong LY, Worthington HV, et al. Fluoride mouthrinses for preventing dental caries in children and adolescents. Cochrane Database Syst Rev 2016;(7):CD002284.
16. Marinho VC, Worthington HV, Walsh T, et al. Fluoride varnishes for preventing dental caries in children and adolescents. Cochrane Database Syst Rev 2013;(7):CD002279.
17. Marinho VC, Worthington HV, Walsh T, et al. Fluoride gels for preventing dental caries in children and adolescents. Cochrane Database Syst Rev 2015;(6):CD002280. https://doi.org/10.1002/14651858.CD002280.pub2. Review.
18. Fontana M. Caries sealing in permanent teeth [Chapter 7]. In: Schwendicke F, editor. Management of deep carious lesions. Springer International Publishing; 2018. p. 93–112.
19. Griffin S, Naavaal S, Scherrer C, et al. School-based dental sealant programs prevent cavities and are cost-effective. Health Aff (Millwood) 2016;35(12): 2233–40.
20. Wright JT, Tampi MP, Graham L, et al. Sealants for preventing and arresting pit-and-fissure occlusal caries in primary and permanent molars: a systematic review of randomized controlled trials- a report from the American Dental Association and the American Academy of Pediatric Dentistry. J Am Dent Assoc 2016; 147(8):631–45.
21. Fontana M, Platt JA, Eckert GJ, et al. Monitoring of caries lesion severity under sealants for 44 months. J Dent Res 2014;93:1070–5.
22. Schwendicke F, Jäger AM, Paris S, et al. Treating pit-and-fissure caries: a systematic review and network meta-analysis. J Dent Res 2015;94(4):522–33.
23. Marsh PD. In sickness and in health-what does the oral microbiome mean to us? an ecological perspective. Adv Dent Res 2018;29(1):60–5.
24. Rethman MP, Beltran-Aguilar ED, Billings RJ, et al. American Dental Association Council on Scientific Affairs Expert Panel on Nonfluoride Caries-Preventive Agents. Nonfluoride caries-preventive agents: executive summary of evidence-based clinical recommendations. J Am Dent Assoc 2011;142(9):1065–71.
25. Santamaría RM, Innes NPT, Machiulskiene V, et al. Alternative caries management options for primary molars: 2.5-year outcomes of a randomised clinical trial. Caries Res 2018;51(6):605–14.
26. Wolff MS, Schenkel AB. The anticaries efficacy of a 1.5% arginine and fluoride toothpaste. Adv Dent Res 2018;29(1):93–7.
27. Gonzalez-Cabezas C, Fernandez CE. Recent advances in remineralization therapies for caries lesions. Adv Dent Res 2018;29(1):55–9.

Surgical Management of Caries Lesions
Selective Removal of Carious Tissues

Andrea G. Ferreira Zandona, DDS, MSD, PhD

KEYWORDS

- Selective caries removal • Dentin • Caries • Restoration • Deep caries

KEY POINTS

- Selective caries removal preserves tooth structure.
- Presence of bacteria underneath as well-sealed restoration does not preclude lesion arrest.
- Understanding dentin demineralization process is crucial to understanding the new paradigm of surgical management of caries lesions.

INTRODUCTION

For centuries, the understanding of dental caries has focused on excising the problem (caries) and restoring the teeth. In fact, restoration of teeth can be found from ancient writings of many populations including Egyptians, Mesopotamians, Israelites, Indians, Chinese, Greeks, Romans, Aztecs, Mayans, Incas, and Arabs.[1] The first full description of restoration of teeth is attributed to Pierre Fauchard in 1728.[1] Although the understanding of dental caries as a disease has come a long way since then, the approach to dental caries management has not changed significantly.

It is well established that dental caries is a biofilm-mediated disease modulated by diet.[2–4] A cariogenic diet can cause dysbiosis in the oral biofilm,[3–6] over time leading to demineralization of exposed hard tooth surfaces. This ongoing process of repeated demineralization at the enamel subsurface level can eventually progress to a collapse of the surface, causing a cavitation in the enamel surface. As the process continues, demineralization of the inorganic phase of the dentin and denaturation and degradation of the organic phase (primarily dentin collagen) result in dentin cavitation.[7] Severe demineralization of dentin results in the exposure of the protein matrix, which is denatured initially by host matrix metalloproteinases (MMPs) and subsequently degraded by MMPs and other bacterial proteases.[7]

Disclosure: The author has currently funding from NIH, CDC, Delta dental and Colgate. she is a consultant for CALCIVIS and Greenmark.
Department of Comprehensive Care, Tufts University School of Dental Medicine, 1 Kneeland Street, Boston, MA 02111, USA
E-mail address: Andrea.Zandona@tufts.edu

Once cavitation occurs, the biofilm has a protected, highly acidic and anaerobic environment ideal for cariogenic bacteria. Thus progression can occur at a faster rate. Although theoretically any caries lesion given the right conditions can be arrested and have progression to larger lesions forestalled, once cavitation occurs, removal of the biofilm is more difficult, and sealing off the cavity by a restorative intervention is usually needed to stop disease progression. Restorative intervention is also often needed to restore tooth to function and aesthetics and support tooth structure integrity independent of the activity status of the carious lesion.

THE CARIES PROCESS IN DENTIN

The effects of the caries process in dentin have conventionally labeled dentin as affected and infected. These terms are not accurate, as bacteria have been found in even sound dentin; they also are not helpful to the clinician, as it is difficult to distinguish what is affected from infected. Traditionally, it was thought that all tissue affected by the dental caries process should be removed, and all surfaces of the cavity should be left in sound, hard dentin, even if that meant placing the pulp at risk of exposure. Current knowledge indicates that carious tissue should be removed selectively with the goal of preserving tooth structure.[8–10] Understating the processes that occur in dentin because of the dental caries process is important to appreciate the recommended selective caries excavation guidelines. In a vital pulp, with adequate blood supply, the pulp–dentin complex reacts to caries activity by attempting to initiate remineralization and blocking off the open tubules. These reactions, which occur even before the lesion has reached the dentin, result from odontoblastic activity[11] and the physical process of demineralization and remineralization. The pulp does not need to be directly exposed to the biofilm to elicit an inflammatory response, as toxins and other metabolic byproducts can penetrate via the dentinal tubules to the pulp. Even when the lesion is limited to enamel, the pulp can be shown to respond with inflammatory cells.[12–14]

Demineralization in dentin occurs at first via weak organic acids which demineralize dentin and expose its organic matrix; the organic matrix, particularly collagen, is then denatured and degraded, eventually losing its structural integrity and being invaded by bacteria.

Initial Stages of Dentin Demineralization

During the initial stages of caries lesions or mild caries activity, as found in slowly advancing caries lesions, a long-term, low-level acid demineralization of dentin occurs. Dentin responds to the stimulus of its first caries demineralization episode by deposition of crystalline material from the intertubular dentin in the lumen of the tubules in the advanced demineralization front (formally called affected dentin). The refractive index of the dentin changes, and the intertubular dentin with more mineral content than normal dentin is termed sclerotic dentin (**Fig. 1**). The apparent function of the sclerotic dentin is to wall off a lesion by blocking (sealing) the tubules. The permeability of sclerotic dentin is greatly reduced compared with that of normal dentin because of the decrease in the tubule lumen diameter.[15] Hypermineralized areas may be seen on radiographs as zones of increased radiopacity (often S-shaped following the course of the tubules) ahead of the advancing, remove portion of the lesion. Sclerotic dentin formation may also be seen under an old restoration. Sclerotic dentin is usually shiny and darker in color but feels hard to the explorer tip (**Fig. 2**). Hard dentin represents the deepest zone of a caries lesion, – assuming the lesion has not yet reached the pulp, and may include tertiary dentin, sclerotic dentin, and normal (or

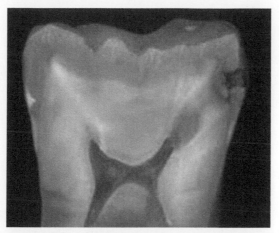

Fig. 1. Transparent dentin visible below sclerotic dentin in a cavitated lesion.

sound) dentin. Clinically this dentin is hard, cannot be easily penetrated with a blunt explorer, and can only be removed by a bur or a sharp cutting instrument. By contrast, normal, freshly cut dentin lacks a shiny, reflective surface and allows some penetration from a sharp explorer tip. When these affected tubules become completely occluded by the mineral precipitate, they appear clear when a histologic section of the tooth is evaluated. This portion of dentin has been termed translucent dentin and is the result of mineral loss in the intertubular dentin and precipitation of this mineral in the tubule lumen. Consequently, translucent dentin is softer than normal dentin[16] and is called firm dentin, in contrast to sound dentin (ie, hard) dentin. Although organic acids attack the mineral and organic contents of dentin, the collagen cross-linking remains intact in this zone and can serve as a template for remineralization of intertubular dentin. Therefore, provided that the pulp remains vital, firm (affected) dentin is remineralizable. Clinically, firm dentin is resistant to hand excavation and can only be removed by exerting pressure. The transition between soft and firm dentin can have a leathery texture, particularly in slowly advancing lesions, and has been called leathery dentin. Clinically, leathery dentin does not deform upon pressure from an instrument but can be excavated with hand instruments such as spoons and curette without much pressure.

Advanced Stages of Dentin Demineralization

More intense caries activity results in bacterial invasion of dentin. The most superficial (closer to the tooth surface) zone of the carious dentin is the necrotic zone.[2] This soft (formerly infected) dentin is primarily characterized by bacterial contamination and contains a wide variety of pathogenic materials or irritants, including high acid levels, hydrolytic enzymes, bacteria, and bacterial cellular debris. These products can cause the degeneration and death of odontoblasts and their tubular extensions below the lesion and a mild inflammation of the pulp. The pulp may be irritated sufficiently from high acid levels or bacterial enzyme production to cause the formation (from undifferentiated mesenchymal cells) of replacement odontoblasts (secondary odontoblasts). These cells produce reparative dentin (reactionary or tertiary dentin) on the affected portion of the pulp chamber wall. This dentin is different from the normal dentinal apposition that occurs throughout the life of the tooth by primary (original) odontoblasts.[17,18] The structure of reparative dentin varies from well-organized tubular dentin (less often) to irregular atubular dentin (more often), depending on the

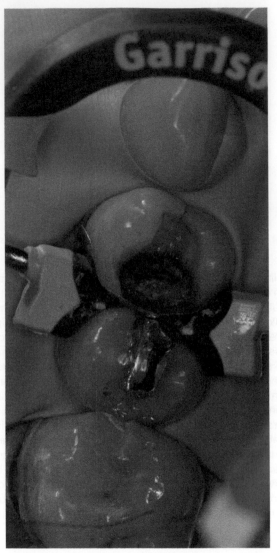

Fig. 2. Sclerotic dentin. Note how the dentin appears shiny and dark. This dentin usually has a firm texture. (*Courtesy of* Oriana Capin, DDS, MSD, Clinical Assistant Professor, Indiana University School of Dentistry.)

severity of the stimulus. Reparative dentin is an effective barrier, allowing limited diffusion of material through the tubules, and is an important step in the repair of dentin. This carious soft dentin closer to the tooth surface has low mineral content, and irreversibly denatured collagen. Histologically, this zone may be referred to as necrotic and contaminated. Although soft dentin typically does not self-repair, the advance front of the soft dentin zone (near firm dentin) is characterized by superficial bacterial invasion, and the caries process can still be stalled when a good restorative seal is obtained. Clinically, soft dentin lacks structure and can be easily excavated with hand and rotary instrumentation (**Fig. 3**).

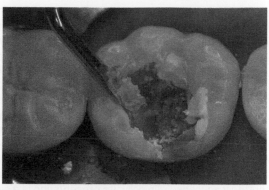

Fig. 3. Soft Dentin. This dentin appears wet and is easily removed with an excavator. It is highly contaminated and cannot be remineralized. (*Courtesy of* Adalberto Vasconcellos.)

The Pulpal Response

The success of dentinal reparative responses, either by remineralization of intertubular dentin and apposition of peritubular dentin or by reparative dentin, depends on the severity of the caries challenge and the ability of the pulp to respond.[19] The pulpal blood supply may be the most important limiting factor to the pulpal responses. Acute, rapidly advancing caries lesions with high levels of acid production overpower host defenses of the pulp and result in infection, abscess, and death of the pulp. Compared with other oral tissues, the pulp is poorly tolerant of inflammation. Small, localized infections in the pulp produce an inflammatory response involving capillary dilation, local edema, and stagnation of blood flow. Because the pulp is contained in a sealed chamber, and its blood is supplied through narrow root canals, any stagnation of blood flow can result in local anoxia and necrosis. The local necrosis leads to more inflammation, edema, and stagnation of blood flow in the immediately adjacent pulp tissue, which becomes necrotic in a cascading process that rapidly spreads to involve the entire pulp.

With the understanding that in a tooth affected by caries there may be different zones in dentin, from the most outer surface, soft, leathery, firm, and hard or sound,[8] the caries excavation can be discussed.

SELECTIVE CARIES EXCAVATION

Traditionally, before placing a restoration, excavation of all tissues affected by caries was recommended. The goal was to have all walls of the cavity on sound, hard dentin. The current understanding of the caries process indicates that preserving tooth structure can lead to better long-term outcomes. Selective caries excavation (SCE) refers to preserving tooth structure by delineating excavation in the pulpal and axial wall according to the lesion severity and depth in a vital tooth with no symptoms or signs of pulpal pathology.[2,8]

Moderate lesions (lesions not reaching the inner one-third of dentin and with no anticipated risk of pulp exposure) should be excavated to a caries-free dentin-enamel junction (DEJ) and firm dentin. Advanced (deep) lesions (lesions reaching the inner one-third of dentin and with anticipated risk of pulp exposure) should be excavated to a caries-free DEJ and soft dentin, following a selective caries removal (SCR) protocol.[8,10,20–22]

There should be some considerations when this protocol is used. The tooth must be deemed restorable, and all peripheral walls need to be prepared to sound DEJ to assure a well-sealed restoration. The pulp must be sensible that is, vital with no symptoms of irreversible pulpitis. SCR consists of caries removal peripherally to a sound, caries-free DEJ; axially and pulpally, caries is removed to within approximately 1 mm of the pulp within soft dentin. A glass ionomer (eg, Fuji IX, GC America, Alsip, Illinois) temporary restoration or a definitive restoration is then placed. Growing evidence suggests that temporization followed by re-entry does not contribute to improved clinical outcomes; therefore, current research supports the placement of a definitive restoration.[23–28] SCR allows a restoration to be placed while avoiding pulpal exposure. Avoiding a pulpal exposure has a great impact on the lifetime prognosis of the tooth and long-term treatment costs.[25] Although the residual dentin thickness cannot be accurately assessed clinically, its preservation is a significant factor in avoiding pulpal distress.[25] For chronic (or slowly advancing lesions), the soft dentin can be removed until the sclerotic, hard dentin is reached. In rapidly advancing lesions, little clinical evidence (as determined by texture or color change) exists to indicate the extent of the soft (infected) dentin. For deep lesions, this lack of clinical evidence may result in an excavation that risks pulp exposure. In a tooth with a deep advanced caries lesion, no history of spontaneous pain, normal responses to thermal stimuli, and a vital pulp, a deliberate, selective caries lesion removal as noted previously may be indicated (**Fig. 4**).[2,8] This procedure is supported by a large body of evidence.[24–27,29–34]

Traditionally, removal of the bacterial infection has been seen as an essential part of all operative procedures. However, even removal of dentin up to hard dentin in deep, advanced caries lesions does not assure a sterile dentin, as bacteria have been found to be present in all dentinal layers in deep caries lesions. Nevertheless, even when bacteria are present, compounding evidence indicates that when a good seal is present, the lesion will arrest.[33–36] Therefore, it is not necessary to remove all of the dentin that has been compromised by the caries process. Although caries detection solutions such as 1% acid red 52 (acid rhodamine B or food red 106) in propylene glycol[37] have been developed to help stain the infected layer, these dyes bind and stain the demineralized dentin matrix and do not stain bacteria exclusively. Complete removal of all stained tooth structure in the preparation, therefore, ultimately leads to significantly larger preparations than the traditional visual-tactile method of evaluating for

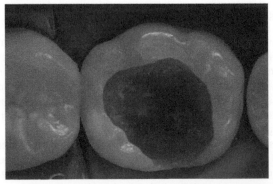

Fig. 4. Selective caries excavation. All margins are on sound tooth structure. Pulpal wall has demineralized dentin. (*Courtesy of* Adalberto Vasconcellos, DDS, MS, PhD, Associate Professor, University of North Carolina at Chapel Hill.)

caries removal, so this is not recommended. Selective caries removal is only indicated on teeth where the restoration will provide a proper seal and all margins will be in a caries-free DEJ.[38–40]

When selective caries removal is performed, it is essential that the patient be well informed. One must consider that radiographically there will be evidence of demineralization underneath the restoration. Additionally, there is a potential of misdiagnosis of pulp vitality, which can cause endodontic complications. There have been advances in vital pulp therapy. Success rates of tricalcium silicates have significantly improved the prognosis of pulp capping and partial and full pulpotomy of permanent mature teeth.[41] Complete caries removal with the option of vital pulp therapy should be an option offered to the patient during the informed consent process.

SUMMARY

SCR is a viable alternative in specific cases to preserve tooth structure while arresting the caries process and restoring tooth to function and esthetics. Proper understanding of the caries process in dentin, case selection, and a meticulously well sealed restoration are vital for success.

REFERENCES

1. Ismail AI, Hasson H, Sohn W. Dental caries in the second millennium. J Dent Educ 2001;65(10):953–9.
2. Ferreira Zandona AG. Dental caries: etiology, clinical characteristics, risk assessment, and management. In: Ritter AV, Boushell L, Walter R, editors. Sturdevant's art and science of operative dentistry. 7 edition. Saint Louis (MO): Elsevier; 2019. p. 40–95.
3. Takahashi N, Nyvad B. Ecological hypothesis of dentin and root caries. Caries Res 2016;50(4):422–31.
4. Takahashi N, Nyvad B. The role of bacteria in the caries process: ecological perspectives. J Dent Res 2011;90(3):294–303.
5. Takahashi N, Nyvad B. Caries ecology revisited: microbial dynamics and the caries process. Caries Res 2008;42(6):409–18.
6. Marsh PD. Dental plaque as a biofilm and a microbial community - implications for health and disease. BMC Oral Health 2006;6(Suppl 1):S14.
7. Chaussain-Miller C, Fioretti F, Goldberg M, et al. The role of matrix metalloproteinases (MMPs) in human caries. J Dent Res 2006;85(1):22–32.
8. Innes NP, Frencken JE, Bjorndal L, et al. Managing carious lesions: consensus recommendations on terminology. Adv Dent Res 2016;28(2):49–57.
9. Innes NP, Frencken JE, Schwendicke F. Don't know, can't do, won't change: barriers to moving knowledge to action in managing the carious lesion. J Dent Res 2016;95(5):485–6.
10. Schwendicke F, Frencken JE, Bjorndal L, et al. Managing carious lesions: consensus recommendations on carious tissue removal. Adv Dent Res 2016; 28(2):58–67.
11. Farges JC, Alliot-Licht B, Renard E, et al. Dental pulp defence and repair mechanisms in dental caries. Mediators Inflamm 2015;2015:230251.
12. Paris S, Wolgin M, Kielbassa AM, et al. Gene expression of human beta-defensins in healthy and inflamed human dental pulps. J Endod 2009;35(4): 520–3.
13. Baume LJ. Dental pulp conditions in relation to carious lesions. Int Dent J 1970; 20(2):309–37.

14. Brannstrom M, Lind PO. Pulpal response to early dental caries. J Dent Res 1965; 44(5):1045–50.
15. Pashley DH. Clinical correlations of dentin structure and function. J Prosthet Dent 1991;66(6):777–81.
16. Ogawa K, Yamashita Y, Ichijo T, et al. The ultrastructure and hardness of the transparent layer of human carious dentin. J Dent Res 1983;62(1):7–10.
17. Bjorndal L. Presence or absence of tertiary dentinogenesis in relation to caries progression. Adv Dent Res 2001;15:80–3.
18. Bjorndal L, Mjor IA. Pulp-dentin biology in restorative dentistry. Part 4. Dental caries–characteristics of lesions and pulpal reactions. Quintessence Int 2001; 32(9):717–36.
19. Bjorndal L. The caries process and its effect on the pulp: the science is changing and so is our understanding. Pediatr Dent 2008;30(3):192–6.
20. Bjorndal L. Buonocore Memorial Lecture. Dentin caries: progression and clinical management. Oper Dent 2002;27(3):211–7.
21. Bjorndal L. Indirect pulp therapy and stepwise excavation. Pediatr Dent 2008; 30(3):225–9.
22. Banerjee A, Frencken JE, Schwendicke F, et al. Contemporary operative caries management: consensus recommendations on minimally invasive caries removal. Br Dent J 2017;223(3):215–22.
23. Oen KT, Thompson VP, Vena D, et al. Attitudes and expectations of treating deep caries: a PEARL Network survey. Gen Dent 2007;55(3):197–203.
24. Pinheiro SL, Simionato MR, Imparato JC, et al. Antibacterial activity of glass-ionomer cement containing antibiotics on caries lesion microorganisms. Am J Dent 2005;18(4):261–6.
25. Ricketts D. Management of the deep carious lesion and the vital pulp dentine complex. Br Dent J 2001;191(11):606–10.
26. Ricketts DN, Kidd EA, Innes N, et al. Complete or ultraconservative removal of de-cayed tissue in unfilled teeth. Cochrane Database Syst Rev 2006;(3):CD003808.
27. van Amerongen WE. Dental caries under glass ionomer restorations. J Public Health Dent 1996;56(3 Spec No):150–4 [discussion: 161–3].
28. Bjorndal L, Kidd EA. The treatment of deep dentine caries lesions. Dent Update 2005;32(7):402–4, 407-410, 413.
29. Ricketts DN, Pitts NB. Novel operative treatment options. Monogr Oral Sci 2009; 21:174–87.
30. Thompson V, Craig RG, Curro FA, et al. Treatment of deep carious lesions by complete excavation or partial removal: a critical review. J Am Dent Assoc 2008;139(6):705–12.
31. Bjorndal L, Larsen T. Changes in the cultivable flora in deep carious lesions following a stepwise excavation procedure. Caries Res 2000;34(6):502–8.
32. Uribe S. Partial caries removal in symptomless teeth reduces the risk of pulp exposure. Evid Based Dent 2006;7(4):94.
33. Maltz M, Garcia R, Jardim JJ, et al. Randomized trial of partial vs. stepwise caries removal: 3-year follow-up. J Dent Res 2012;91(11):1026–31.
34. Alves LS, Fontanella V, Damo AC, et al. Qualitative and quantitative radiographic assessment of sealed carious dentin: a 10-year prospective study. Oral Surg Oral Med Oral Pathol Oral Radiol Endod 2010;109(1):135–41.
35. Lima KC, Coelho LT, Pinheiro IV, et al. Microbiota of dentinal caries as assessed by reverse-capture checkerboard analysis. Caries Res 2011;45(1):21–30.
36. Banerjee A, Kidd EA, Watson TF. In vitro evaluation of five alternative methods of carious dentine excavation. Caries Res 2000;34(2):144–50.

37. Fusayama T. Two layers of carious dentin; diagnosis and treatment. Oper Dent 1979;4(2):63–70.
38. Hamama HH, Yiu CK, Burrow MF, et al. Systematic review and meta-analysis of randomized clinical trials on chemomechanical caries removal. Oper Dent 2015;40(4):E167–78.
39. Hamama HH, Yiu CK, Burrow MF, et al. Chemical, morphological and microhardness changes of dentine after chemomechanical caries removal. Aust Dent J 2013;58(3):283–92.
40. Corralo DJ, Maltz M. Clinical and ultrastructural effects of different liners/restorative materials on deep carious dentin: a randomized clinical trial. Caries Res 2013;47(3):243–50.
41. Hoefler V, Nagaoka H, Miller CS. Long-term survival and vitality outcomes of permanent teeth following deep caries treatment with step-wise and partial-caries-removal: a systematic review. J Dent 2016;54:25–32.

Performance of Adhesives and Restorative Materials After Selective Removal of Carious Lesions
Restorative Materials with Anticaries Properties

Leo Tjäderhane, DDS, PhD[a,b,*], Arzu Tezvergil-Mutluay, DDS, PhD[c]

KEYWORDS

- Amalgam • Composite resin • Glass ionomer • Calcium silicates • Carious dentin

KEY POINTS

- Carious dentin can be left under provisional or permanent restoration without risk of caries progression.
- Restoration marginal sealing must be tight and placed on intact enamel and dentin.
- There is little evidence of any contemporary restorative material to be superior as temporary or permanent filling over carious dentin.
- Cavity lining is not necessary for pulpal health or dentin remineralization.

INTRODUCTION

With the advances in understanding the biofilm and improvements in the material and bonding technologies, the conventional concept of complete caries removal combined with extension into sound tissue for prevention was replaced with the minimal invasive selective or stepwise carious tissue-removal approach. The advent of selective removal of carious tissue has raised a question: which restorative materials should be used over carious tissue left under the restoration? Before discussing the performance of restorative materials, it is essential to realize that the approach to leave at least firm

Disclosure: The authors have nothing to disclose.
[a] Department of Oral and Maxillofacial Diseases, University of Helsinki, Helsinki University Hospital, PO Box 41, Helsinki 00014, Finland; [b] Research Unit of Oral Health Sciences, Medical Research Center Oulu (MRC Oulu), Oulu University Hospital, University of Oulu, Oulu, Finland; [c] Department of Cariology and Restorative Dentistry, Adhesive Dentistry Research Group, Institute of Dentistry, Turku University Hospital, TYKS, University of Turku, Lemminkäisenkatu 2, Turku 20520, Finland
* Corresponding author. Department Oral and Maxillofacial Diseases, University of Helsinki, PO Box 41, Helsinki 00014, Finland.
E-mail address: Leo.Tjaderhane@helsinki.fi

Dent Clin N Am 63 (2019) 715–729
https://doi.org/10.1016/j.cden.2019.05.001
0011-8532/19/© 2019 Elsevier Inc. All rights reserved.

caries-affected dentin under the restoration is not necessarily new. Lesion in dentin does not have a distinct border between carious and healthy tissue, and judgment between "carious" and completely "healthy" dentin is clinically challenging if not impossible. Even with nonselective caries removal, some firm caries-affected dentin is left behind, as visual-tactile diagnosis of residual caries is very subjective method,[1] and even the organic component of dentin may be altered in early phases of dentinal caries.[2] The amount of caries-affected or caries-infected dentin left behind depends also on the method used for caries removal.[3,4] It may thus be argued that clinicians have been practicing selective removal of carious tissue to reach firm or even leathery dentin even in the era when the nonselective "complete" caries removal was a must.

The choice of restorative material is affected by the carious tissue-removal approach: is the tooth permanently restored, or is stepwise carious tissue removal chosen to avoid pulp perforation and retain pulp vitality? If permanent restoration is placed immediately, clinical features such as the remaining coronal tooth tissue, the size of the restoration, occlusal forces, caries risk, and esthetics affect the material selection. This applies especially to carious tissue removal extended to firm dentin. If leathery dentin, which does not deform under pressure but is still relatively easily removed with an excavator, is left underneath, the clinician may also want to consider how this type of suboptimal tooth substrate may affect the behavior and longevity of the restoration. In addition, the location of the lesion and remaining carious tissue may significantly affect the long-term outcome of the restoration. It should be emphasized here that selective removal applies only to dentin facing the pulp: all carious enamel and soft-leathery dentin should always be removed from the cavity margins to ensure restoration placement to structurally and mechanically strong enamel[5,6] (**Fig. 1**) and to ensure a tight marginal seal.

STEPWISE REMOVAL OF CARIOUS DENTIN

Stepwise removal refers to two-step carious tissue removal, whereby in the first stage, selective removal is extended to soft dentin in the pulpal side and the cavity is sealed

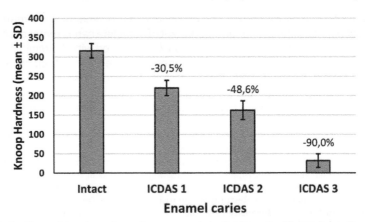

Fig. 1. Reduction of hardness in carious enamel, indicating significant loss of mechanical strength with the advance of demineralization according to the International Caries Detection and Assessment System (ICDAS) classification. The percentages above the bars show the actual loss of hardness compared with sound enamel. (*Data from* Shimizu A, Yamamoto T, Nakashima S, et al. Measurement of surface hardness of primary carious lesions in extracted human enamel -measurement of Knoop hardness using Cariotester. Dent Mater J 2015;34:252–6.)

with a long-temporary restoration for 6 to 12 months. At control, the cavity is re-entered to remove the remaining soft carious tissue and place permanent restoration. The stepwise approach is particularly useful in deep lesions where the risk for pulp exposure with selective carious tissue removal is imminent.[7–11]

The Use of Liners During Stepwise Removal of Carious Dentin

Cavity liners have been promoted at the pulpal walls in deep cavities to reduce hypersensitivity, kill bacteria, block the harmful components of the restorative materials from reaching the pulp, induce reactionary dentin formation, and/or promote remineralization. Calcium hydroxide (CaOH) especially has a long history as a lining material under restorations, including the early stepwise excavation studies. A systematic review concluded that CaOH is effective in reducing bacteria and promoting remineralization of remaining carious dentin.[12] However, the review included 13 studies, of which 6 had no control group, 2 had CaOH in the control group, and 2 did not have CaOH in either experimental or control groups. More recent studies have indicated that the use of CaOH or any other contemporary liner material does not have a significant effect on the clinical or microbial outcome.[13–20] Another systematic review and meta-analysis found no difference in pulpal response between CaOH and resin-modified glass-ionomer liners.[21] Thus, the available evidence does not support the use of liners if good marginal seal of the cavity is achieved.

However, CaOH may have stronger antibacterial effects than other commonly used lining materials, and may reduce bacterial numbers much more effectively than only sealing the cavity.[17] In the case of stepwise excavation close to the pulp, when remaining soft dentin is apparently heavily infected it may be advisable to use CaOH liner not only to reduce bacterial load but also to help prevent the accidental pulpal perforation during the re-entry, especially when tooth-colored materials are used as temporary filling.

Restorative Material During Stepwise Removal of Carious Dentin

Numerous materials have been used as temporary restorations in stepwise removal studies,[12,22] and there is no apparent consensus of one material being superior to others. The requirements for the temporary restorative material are tight seal, sufficient longevity, and ease of removal during re-entry. Early studies with shorter follow-up time (usually 3 months or less) used zinc oxide-eugenol-based materials.[12] However, the currently recommended 6- to 12-month follow-up time may require more durable material to ensure a marginal seal. Amalgam has a good longevity and is especially successful in patients at high risk of caries.[23,24] The corrosion products seal the margin soon after placement, and antibacterial properties may protect against secondary carious lesions. Amalgam is also easy to discriminate from tooth tissue during removal, but poor aesthetics and increasing limitations for the use of mercury-containing materials and procedures (Minimata Convention on Mercury: http://mercuryconvention.org/) are limiting the use of dental amalgam worldwide. High-viscosity glass-ionomer cements (HV-GICs) have good biocompatibility, bond chemically to dental hard tissues, release fluoride, may protect against secondary caries, and have good longevity especially in class I and II cavities.[25,26] Being less aesthetic than composite resin, it is easier to remove during re-entry, but still much more aesthetic than amalgam. Composite resins form a tight seal in cavity margins, but bonding to carious dentin, especially to soft carious dentin, is poor[27–30] (**Figs. 2 and 3**), and the alterations of mechanical properties in caries-affected dentin[31,32] may subject dentin to cohesive damage caused by composite resin shrinkage stress[33] (see **Fig. 3**). In addition, placing composite resin requires more time, and because of

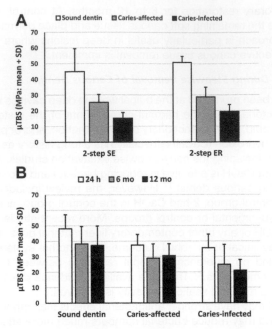

Fig. 2. (*A*) Comparison of immediate bond strength of 2-step self-etch adhesive (2-step SE) and 2-step etch-and-rinse adhesive (2-step ER). (*B*) Comparison of immediate, 6-month, and 12-month bond strength of a 2-step self-etch adhesive. μTBS, microtensile bond strength. (*Data from* [*A*] Yoshiyama M, Tay FR, Doi J, et al. Bonding of self-etch and total-etch adhesives to carious dentin. J Dent Res 2002;81:556–60; and [*B*] Costa AR, Garcia-Godoy F, Correr-Sobrinho L, et al. Influence of different dentin substrate (caries-affected, caries-infected, sound) on long-term μTBS. Braz Dent J 2017;28:16–23.)

the tight bond to sound marginal dentin and enamel and good aesthetics, the loss of sound tissue may occur during re-entry. In conclusion, HV-GIC is the material of choice for a long-term provisional restoration in stepwise removal of carious dentin.

SELECTIVE REMOVAL OF CARIOUS TISSUE

Selective removal of carious tissue may reach firm or leathery dentin, or can be left to soft (caries-infected) dentin.[34] In very shallow lesions, removal to firm dentin may be necessary to reach the required thickness of the restorative material. In moderately deep cavities, relatively hard but leathery dentin can be left to the pulpal cavity side to avoid pulpal perforation. Clinical studies have indicated that vitality is retained with selective carious tissue removal in both primary and permanent teeth.[35–39]

Remineralization of the partially demineralized carious dentin, reaching the original hardness and mechanical properties, is the ultimate goal of the restorative material research, but is not easy to achieve. The mechanical properties of mineralized dentin depend highly on intrafibrillar minerals, and true remineralization should aim at re-establishing intrafibrillar minerals.[2] This, however, may be a difficult if not impossible task with the contemporary materials[40] if the original nucleation site phosphoproteins have been lost at the space between the collagen molecules where the intrafibrillar mineral is sited (the gap area),[2] and plain rehardening is still the best achievable goal.

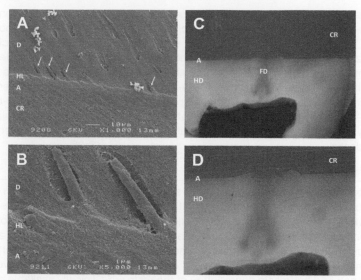

Fig. 3. The intimate contact of adhesive-bound composite resin restoration with Single Bond 1 adhesive to sound dentin. (*A*) Approximately 5-μm thick hybrid layer (HL), containing exposed collagen and adhesive resin, creates the bond between the adhesive layer (A) and dentin (D). *Arrows* indicate resin plugs penetrating into dentinal tubules. CR, composite resin (scanning electron microscopy, original magnification ×1000). (*B*) Higher magnification of the hybrid layer (HL) and resin plugs, mostly separated from the dentinal tubule walls and not contributing to the bond except at the tubule orifice (*asterisk*) where the acid etching has exposed the collagen. A, adhesive layer; D, dentin (scanning electron microscopy, original magnification ×5000). (*C*) Composite resin restoration built over flat dentin surface and cut into 1-mm slices. At the site of caries-affected firm dentin (FD) a gap in the adhesive interface is observed, as well as cohesive fracture lines surrounding the caries-affected dentin, presumably caused by polymerization shrinkage and stress and impacted by the lower mechanical properties of carious dentin (stereomicroscopy, original magnification ×20). HD, hard (sound) dentin. (*D*) Higher magnification (×32) of the firm caries-affected dentin shown in (*C*).

Similar to stepwise removal of carious dentin already discussed, there are no clinical studies or consensus of the best restorative material over the caries-affected— leathery or firm—dentin. The advantages and disadvantages of contemporary direct restorative materials are now discussed in relation to caries.

Amalgam

Amalgam and composite resins are the most common "permanent" direct restoration materials globally. Recent meta-analysis indicated that amalgam restorations still have better longevity than composite resin restorations.[41,42] However, it should be noted that most of the studies included in the meta-analysis were relatively old, excluding the advances in composite resin restorative materials and techniques. It should also be noted that traditionally nonselective caries removal to hard dentin has been practiced, and little is known of the effect on survival of leathery/firm caries-affected dentin left underneath on purpose during amalgam restorations.

Amalgam corrosion products seal the gap between the tooth tissue and restoration, and antibacterial properties of amalgam have been held responsible for the protection against secondary carious lesions. However, the corrosion products may also affect caries-affected dentin. Along with tin, zinc is consistently found under amalgam fillings in caries-affected dentin and in artificially demineralized dentin exposed to amalgam.[43,44] Zinc-containing amalgams decrease the microleakage much faster than nonzinc amalgams,[45] excess of zinc effectively inhibits collagen-degrading matrix metalloproteinases (MMPs) participating in the dentinal caries process and adhesive hybrid layer degradation,[2,33] and Zn-containing amalgams promote remineralization and increase nanomechanical properties of subjacent caries-affected dentin.[46–49] It is tempting to speculate that zinc anticollagenolytic/remineralizing effects may contribute to the longevity of amalgam restorations placed over caries-affected dentin.

Composite Resin

As mentioned earlier, the immediate bond strength to caries-affected dentin is lower than to sound dentin[30] and even lower with caries-infected dentin[27–29] (see **Fig. 2**). The literature also indicates that etch-and-rinse adhesives may yield somewhat higher bond strength than self-etch materials to caries-affected dentin.[30] In addition, dentin bond strength decreases with time regardless of the type of dentin (see **Fig. 2**), mainly because of collagenolytic enzymes degrading the adhesive hybrid layer collagen and hydrolytic degradation of the resin.[2,33] Clinically available methods to achieve collagenolytic enzyme inhibition and improve bond-strength durability include cavity pretreatment with chlorhexidine and the use of quaternary ammonium methacrylate (QAM)-containing materials.[33,50] QAMs, such as 12-methacryloyloxy-dodecylpyridinium bromide (MDPB), present in some clinically available adhesives, are polymerizable antimicrobial compounds and the most versatile, most studied, and perhaps most promising adhesive resin components with antibacterial properties.[51] In addition, they also inhibit dentin MMPs,[52,53] which has been indicated as a potential reason for prolonged durability of dentin bonding in vitro.[54] Despite very promising in vitro and in vivo experimental results, the evidence of improvement in clinical conditions is still lacking.[55–57] The use of noncarious cervical lesions instead of carious lesions and the still short follow-up times may have contributed to the results of the clinical studies. Therefore clinically, bonding to caries-affected and especially caries-infected dentin can only be recommended if the area is very limited and the peripheral seal of the cavity is placed on sound dentin and enamel to ensure a durable bonding.

Cariogenic bacteria, such as Streptococcus mutans, readily accumulate on the surface of composite resin, and improving the antimicrobial properties of the restorative or adhesive materials is an attractive alternative both to reduce the adverse effects of bacteria remaining under the restoration and to reduce secondary caries. Demineralization is not the only mechanism whereby bacteria may accelerate secondary caries at the interface. Cariogenic bacteria possess esterase activity in levels that can degrade resin composites and adhesives,[58–61] and degradation products may further increase the expression of the esterase and accelerate the biodegradation of the restoration components.[62] Several attempts have been made to introduce antimicrobial biofilm-modulating properties of composite restorative materials,[61,63,64] but there is very little evidence of clinical benefits of these materials.[63,65]

Glass-Ionomer Cements

Fluoride-releasing materials—GICs, resin-modified GICs (RM-GICs), and compomers, are promoted as cariostatic restorative materials and as an alternative to composite or amalgam restorations. Although the fluoride release of RM-GIC and compomer is significantly lower than of GIC[66] (**Fig. 4**) and has not been shown to have any

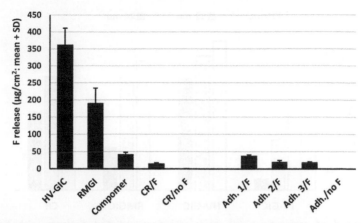

Fig. 4. Cumulative fluoride release of different restorative materials in clinical use. Adh., adhesive; CR, composite resin; HV-GIC, high-viscosity glass-ionomer cement; RMGI, resin-modified glass-ionomer cement. (*Data from* Dionysopoulos D, Koliniotou-Koumpia E, Helvatzoglou-Antoniades M, et al. Fluoride release and recharge abilities of contemporary fluoride-containing restorative materials and dental adhesives. Dent Mater J 2013;32:296–304.)

significant effect, there is emerging support for the therapeutic effect of GIC against caries,[67] especially for HV-GIC.[26] Meta-analyses indicate a clinical caries-preventive effect of GIC, but because of the lack of randomized controlled studies the results are limited to comparison with amalgam and single-surface fillings in permanent teeth.[26,68] Unlike contemporary adhesives, which have a significantly lower bond strength to caries-affected dentin than sound dentin regardless of the adhesive system used[30] (see **Fig. 2**), HV-GICs have similar bond strength to both normal and caries-affected dentin.[69] El-Deeb and Mobarak[69] concluded that HV-GICs can be recommended to restore cavities after selective removal of carious dentin.

Postirradiation xerostomic patients present very high caries rates, and provide an ideal population for investigating the effects of restorative material in a reduced time frame.[70] Several studies have demonstrated good survival rates for HV-GICs in these patients (**Fig. 5**). More notably, both low-viscosity GIC (LV-GIC) and HV-GIC restorations completely prevented secondary caries even in patients with low compliance to fluoride use or when the restoration was completely lost,[70–73] and the deteriorated restorations could also be turned into sandwich restorations.

van de Sande and colleagues[74] studied the clinical survival of posterior class I–II composite resin restorations with and without GIC as base for up to 18 years. The data demonstrated markedly better survival rates with the GIC base up to 15 years (**Fig. 6**). Even better survival of GIC-based sandwich restorations was observed in a similar study, with 92.6% and 82.4% survival after 10 and 18 years, respectively.[75] The effect may be related to decreased polymerization shrinkage stress in large mesio-occlusal-distal (MOD) cavities,[76] as RM-GIC lining does not improve survival.[14,77] On the contrary, 9-year survival of 88.1% for composite resin without RM-GIC lining and 70.5% with RM-GIC lining were observed.[77]

The reputation of poor clinical performance of GIC restorations may be based on the LV-GICs that may already be considered old-fashioned materials. Contemporary HV-GICs have recorded much higher survival rates, even on the occlusion-bearing surfaces (**Fig. 7**). Scholtanus and Huysmans[25] followed 116 class II GIC restorations

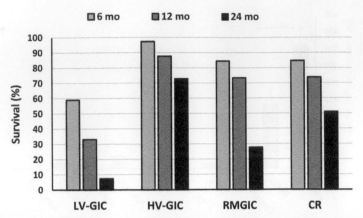

Fig. 5. Survival of restorations in xerostomic postirradiated patients with head and neck cancer. CR, composite resin; HV-GIC, high-viscosity glass-ionomer cement; LV-GIC, low-viscosity glass-ionomer cement; RMGIC, resin-modified glass-ionomer cement. (*Data from* Refs.[70–73])

(Fuji IX; GC Corp, Tokyo, Japan) for 7 years. No failures were observed within the first 18 months, and at the end of the evaluation period 63% survived (**Fig. 8**). All but one failure was due to loss of restorative material in the proximal area, leading to loss of interproximal contact easily reparable to a sandwich restoration. The results were supported by another study reporting 96% survival during a shorter (24 months) follow-up.[78]

Recent systematic review indicated that there is no difference in failure rates between HV-GIC and hybrid resin composite restorations, and the superiority claims

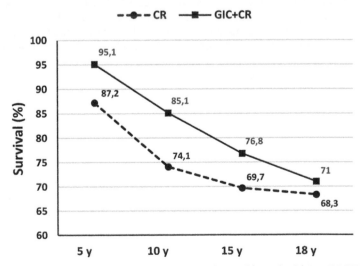

Fig. 6. Survival of class I–II composite resin restorations with and without LV-GIC base. CR, composite resin. (*Data from* van de Sande FH, Rodolpho PA, Basso GR, et al. 18-year survival of posterior composite resin restorations with and without glass ionomer cement as base. Dent Mater 2015;31:669–75.)

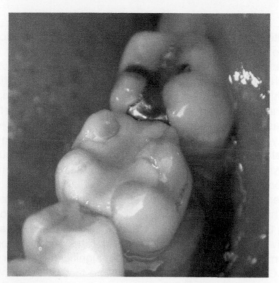

Fig. 7. High-viscosity glass-ionomer cement MOD restoration in lower first molar after more than 11 years in service.

of direct resin composite restorations in single or multisurface cavities in posterior permanent teeth cannot be justified by the current poor clinical evidence.[79] However, in most studies the follow-up time was reasonably short. Despite the improvement in formulations, GICs still have lower mechanical properties compared with composites, are less aesthetic, and are prone to faster degradation in the erosive environment.[80]

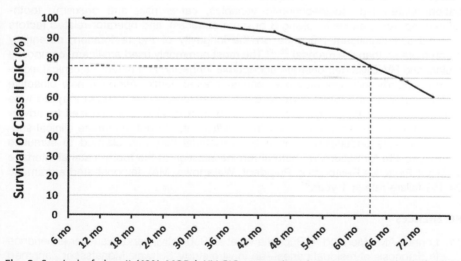

Fig. 8. Survival of class II (40% MODs) HV-GIC restorations in permanent molars of adult patients in general practice. Five-year survival was still slightly more than 75% (*dashed line*). (*Data from* Scholtanus JD, Huysmans MC. Clinical failure of class-II restorations of a highly viscous glass-ionomer material over a 6-year period: a retrospective study. J Dent 2007;35:156–62.)

Calcium Silicates

Unlike other contemporary restorative materials, the hydraulic calcium silicate cements Biodentine (Septodont, St.-Maur-des-Fossés, France) and mineral trioxide cement (MTA)-based products promote the release of signaling molecules from the dentin underneath and elicit a physiologic response from the host tissue, leading to tissue repair.[81] Although MTA may be excellent for direct pulp capping, as a base material Biodentine has better mechanical properties (compressive and flexural strength, hardness, and elastic modulus) and high release of calcium.[82] Unlike with GIC, tooth discoloration may still be a matter of concern, even though not as much as with MTA.[82] Low initial bond strength,[83] increase in compressive strength, and decrease in microleakage with time[84] underline the importance of allowing full maturation before placing the composite over the Biodentine base.[82]

Although Biodentine has demonstrated successful outcomes in a variety of treatment scenarios, high-quality clinical trials are still scarce.[82] In a prospective clinical study comparing Biodentine and HV-GIC (Fuji IX) placed over caries-affected dentin in a closed-sandwich model, the clinical success rates after 12 months were equal (83.3% for both materials)[85] and slightly but not significantly better with Biodentine (77.8%) than for GIC (66.7%) at 24 months.[86] More teeth with a new or progressing periapical lesion detected with cone-beam computed tomography at 12 months occurred in teeth restored with GIC, but there were more nonvital teeth and teeth with severe preoperative symptoms in the GIC group at the onset of the study.[85] Thus, the role of material in endodontic complications remains to be demonstrated. If Biodentine is left uncovered for a longer time, the increase in deficiencies in marginal adaptation may require a close follow-up.[87]

SUMMARY

Regardless of the restorative material, secondary caries and fractures are the main reasons for failures.[41,88,89] For the material selection for an individual tooth, patient-related (eg, socioeconomic variables, caries risk, and bruxism), tooth-related (eg, restorations involving 3 or more surfaces), and operator-related factors may have a significant influence on the longevity of the restoration, potentially much more so than the material.[88,89] The most commonly used amalgam, composite resins, and HV-GICs demonstrate acceptable longevity, and extensive clinical experience supports their use also over caries-affected dentin. Although new bioactive materials may in the future provide even better results, the clinician may be wise to be cautious, as the terms "bioactive" or "biomineralizing" are overused for advertising purposes,[90] and even convincing in vitro data do not guarantee clinical success. This was underlined when a base material that was claimed to stimulate hydroxyapatite formation and natural remineralization at the tooth-material interface (ACTIVA Bioactive Restorative; Pulpdent, Watertown, MA) demonstrated a dramatic 24.1% failure rate in 1 year.[91]

REFERENCES

1. Lennon AM, Wiegand A, Buchalla W, et al. Subjectivity and examiner experience in diagnosis of residual caries—an in vitro study. Schweiz Monatsschr Zahnmed 2007;117:123-7.
2. Tjäderhane L, Buzalaf MA, Carrilho M, et al. Matrix metalloproteinases and other matrix proteinases in relation to cariology: the era of 'dentin degradomics'. Caries Res 2015;49:193-208.

3. Banerjee A, Kidd EA, Watson TF. In vitro evaluation of five alternative methods of carious dentine excavation. Caries Res 2000;34:144–50.

4. Banerjee A, Kidd EA, Watson TF. Scanning electron microscopic observations of human dentine after mechanical caries excavation. J Dent 2000;28:179–86.

5. Huang TT, He LH, Darendeliler MA, et al. Nano-indentation characterisation of natural carious white spot lesions. Caries Res 2010;44:101–7.

6. Shimizu A, Yamamoto T, Nakashima S, et al. Measurement of surface hardness of primary carious lesions in extracted human enamel -measurement of Knoop hardness using Cariotester. Dent Mater J 2015;34:252–6.

7. Leksell E, Ridell K, Cvek M, et al. Pulp exposure after stepwise versus direct complete excavation of deep carious lesions in young posterior permanent teeth. Endod Dent Traumatol 1996;12:192–6.

8. Bjørndal L, Larsen T, Thylstrup A. A clinical and microbiological study of deep carious lesions during stepwise excavation using long treatment intervals. Caries Res 1997;31:411–7.

9. Bjørndal L, Reit C, Bruun G, et al. Treatment of deep caries lesions in adults: randomized clinical trials comparing stepwise vs. direct complete excavation, and direct pulp capping vs. partial pulpotomy. Eur J Oral Sci 2010;118:290–7.

10. Bjørndal L, Fransson H, Bruun G, et al. Randomized clinical trials on deep carious lesions: 5-year follow-up. J Dent Res 2017;96:747–53.

11. Orhan AI, Oz FT, Orhan K. Pulp exposure occurrence and outcomes after 1- or 2-visit indirect pulp therapy vs complete caries removal in primary and permanent molars. Pediatr Dent 2010;32:347–55.

12. Hayashi M, Fujitani M, Yamaki C, et al. Ways of enhancing pulp preservation by stepwise excavation—a systematic review. J Dent 2011;39:95–107.

13. Duque C, Negrini Tde C, Sacono NT, et al. Clinical and microbiological performance of resin-modified glass-ionomer liners after incomplete dentine caries removal. Clin Oral Investig 2009;13:465–71.

14. Banomyong D, Messer H. Two-year clinical study on postoperative pulpal complications arising from the absence of a glass-ionomer lining in deep occlusal resin-composite restorations. J Investig Clin Dent 2013;4:265–70.

15. Corralo DJ, Maltz M. Clinical and ultrastructural effects of different liners/restorative materials on deep carious dentin: a randomized clinical trial. Caries Res 2013;47:243–50.

16. Kuhn E, Chibinski AC, Reis A, et al. The role of glass ionomer cement on the remineralization of infected dentin: an in vivo study. Pediatr Dent 2014;36:E118–24.

17. Schwendicke F, Tu YK, Hsu LY, et al. Antibacterial effects of cavity lining: a systematic review and network meta-analysis. J Dent 2015;43:1298–307.

18. Opal S, Garg S, Sharma D, et al. In vivo effect of calcium hydroxide and resin-modified glass ionomer cement on carious dentin in young permanent molars: an ultrastructural and macroscopic study. Pediatr Dent 2017;39:1–8.

19. Pereira MA, Santos-Júnior RBD, Tavares JA, et al. No additional benefit of using a calcium hydroxide liner during stepwise caries removal: a randomized clinical trial. J Am Dent Assoc 2017;148:369–76.

20. da Rosa WL, Lima VP, Moraes RR, et al. Is a calcium hydroxide liner necessary in the treatment of deep caries lesions? A systematic review and meta-analysis. Int Endod J 2019;52(5):588–603.

21. Mickenautsch S, Yengopal V, Banerjee A. Pulp response to resin-modified glass ionomer and calcium hydroxide cements in deep cavities: a quantitative systematic review. Dent Mater 2010;26:761–70.

22. Bjørndal L, Thylstrup A. A practice-based study on stepwise excavation of deep carious lesions in permanent teeth: a 1-year follow-up study. Community Dent Oral Epidemiol 1998;26:122–8.
23. Opdam NJ, Bronkhorst EM, Loomans BA, et al. 12-year survival of composite vs. amalgam restorations. J Dent Res 2010;89:1063–7.
24. Kopperud SE, Tveit AB, Gaarden T, et al. Longevity of posterior dental restorations and reasons for failure. Eur J Oral Sci 2012;120:539–48.
25. Scholtanus JD, Huysmans MC. Clinical failure of class-II restorations of a highly viscous glass-ionomer material over a 6-year period: a retrospective study. J Dent 2007;35:156–62.
26. Mickenautsch S. High-viscosity glass-ionomer cements for direct posterior tooth restorations in permanent teeth: the evidence in brief. J Dent 2016;55:121–3.
27. Yoshiyama M, Tay FR, Doi J, et al. Bonding of self-etch and total-etch adhesives to carious dentin. J Dent Res 2002;81:556–60.
28. Yoshiyama M, Tay FR, Torii Y, et al. Resin adhesion to carious dentin. Am J Dent 2003;16:47–52.
29. Costa AR, Garcia-Godoy F, Correr-Sobrinho L, et al. Influence of different dentin substrate (caries-affected, caries-infected, sound) on long-term μTBS. Braz Dent J 2017;28:16–23.
30. Isolan CP, Sarkis-Onofre R, Lima GS, et al. Bonding to sound and caries-affected dentin: a systematic review and meta-analysis. J Adhes Dent 2018;20:7–18.
31. Angker L, Nijhof N, Swain MV, et al. Influence of hydration and mechanical characterization of carious primary dentine using an ultra-micro indentation system (UMIS). Eur J Oral Sci 2004;112:231–6.
32. Ito S, Saito T, Tay FR, et al. Water content and apparent stiffness of non-carious versus caries-affected human dentin. J Biomed Mater Res B Appl Biomater 2005;72:109–16.
33. Tjäderhane L. Dentin bonding: can we make it last? Oper Dent 2015;40:4–18.
34. Schwendicke F, Frencken JE, Bjørndal L, et al. Managing carious lesions: consensus recommendations on carious tissue removal. Adv Dent Res 2016; 28:58–67.
35. Maltz M, Alves LS, Jardim JJ, et al. Incomplete caries removal in deep lesions: a 10-year prospective study. Am J Dent 2011;24:211–4.
36. Maltz M, Jardim JJ, Mestrinho HD, et al. Partial removal of carious dentine: a multicenter randomized controlled trial and 18-month follow-up results. Caries Res 2013;47:103–9.
37. Lenzi TL, Pires CW, Soares FZM, et al. Performance of universal adhesive in primary molars after selective removal of carious tissue: an 18-month randomized clinical trial. Pediatr Dent 2017;39:371–6.
38. Elhennawy K, Finke C, Paris S, et al. Selective vs stepwise removal of deep carious lesions in primary molars: 12-months results of a randomized controlled pilot trial. J Dent 2018;77:72–7.
39. Mello B, Stafuzza T, Vitor L, et al. Evaluation of dentin-pulp complex response after conservative clinical procedures in primary teeth. Int J Clin Pediatr Dent 2018; 11:188–92.
40. Sauro S, Pashley DH. Strategies to stabilise dentine-bonded interfaces through remineralising operative approaches—state of the art. Int J Adhes Adhes 2016; 69:39–57.
41. Rasines Alcaraz MG, Veitz-Keenan A, Sahrmann P, et al. Direct composite resin fillings versus amalgam fillings for permanent or adult posterior teeth. Cochrane Database Syst Rev 2014;(3):CD005620.

42. Moraschini V, Fai CK, Alto RM, et al. Amalgam and resin composite longevity of posterior restorations: a systematic review and meta-analysis. J Dent 2015;43: 1043–50.

43. Kurosaki N, Fusayama T. Penetration of elements from amalgam into dentin. J Dent Res 1973;52:309–17.

44. Scholtanus JD, Ozcan M, Huysmans MC. Penetration of amalgam constituents into dentine. J Dent 2009;37:366–73.

45. Mahler DB, Pham BV, Adey JD. Corrosion sealing of amalgam restorations in vitro. Oper Dent 2009;34:312–20.

46. Toledano M, Aguilera FS, Osorio E, et al. Mechanical and chemical characterisation of demineralised human dentine after amalgam restorations. J Mech Behav Biomed Mater 2015;47:65–76.

47. Toledano M, Aguilera FS, Osorio E, et al. On modeling and nanoanalysis of caries-affected dentin surfaces restored with Zn-containing amalgam and in vitro oral function. Biointerphases 2015;10:041004.

48. Toledano M, Aguilera FS, López-López MT, et al. Zinc-containing restorations create amorphous biogenic apatite at the carious dentin interface: a X-ray diffraction (XRD) crystal lattice analysis. Microsc Microanal 2016;22:1034–46.

49. Toledano M, Osorio E, Aguilera FS, et al. Stored potential energy increases and elastic properties alterations are produced after restoring dentin with Zn-containing amalgams. J Mech Behav Biomed Mater 2018;91:109–21.

50. Breschi L, Maravic T, Cunha SR, et al. Dentin bonding systems: from dentin collagen structure to bond preservation and clinical applications. Dent Mater 2018;34:78–96.

51. Makvandi P, Jamaledin R, Jabbari M, et al. Antibacterial quaternary ammonium compounds in dental materials: a systematic review. Dent Mater 2018;34:851–67.

52. Tezvergil-Mutluay A, Agee KA, Uchiyama T, et al. The inhibitory effects of quaternary ammonium methacrylates on soluble and matrix-bound MMPs. J Dent Res 2011;90:535–40.

53. Tezvergil-Mutluay A, Agee KA, Mazzoni A, et al. Can quaternary ammonium methacrylates inhibit matrix MMPs and cathepsins? Dent Mater 2015;31:e25–32.

54. Tjäderhane L, Nascimento FD, Breschi L, et al. Strategies to prevent hydrolytic degradation of the hybrid layer-A review. Dent Mater 2013;29:999–1011.

55. Sartori N, Stolf SC, Silva SB, et al. Influence of chlorhexidine digluconate on the clinical performance of adhesive restorations: a 3-year follow-up. J Dent 2013;41: 1188–95.

56. Pinto CF, Berger SB, Cavalli V, et al. In situ antimicrobial activity and inhibition of secondary caries of self-etching adhesives containing an antibacterial agent and/ or fluoride. Am J Dent 2015;28:167–73.

57. Favetti M, Schroeder T, Montagner AF, et al. Effectiveness of pre-treatment with chlorhexidine in restoration retention: a 36-month follow-up randomized clinical trial. J Dent 2017;60:44–9.

58. Bourbia M, Ma D, Cvitkovitch DG, et al. Cariogenic bacteria degrade dental resin composites and adhesives. J Dent Res 2013;92:989–94.

59. Huang B, Cvitkovitch DG, Santerre JP, et al. Biodegradation of resin-dentin interfaces is dependent on the restorative material, mode of adhesion, esterase or MMP inhibition. Dent Mater 2018;34:1253–62.

60. Huang B, Siqueira WL, Cvitkovitch DG, et al. Esterase from a cariogenic bacterium hydrolyzes dental resins. Acta Biomater 2018;71:330–8.

61. Stewart CA, Finer Y. Biostable, antidegradative and antimicrobial restorative systems based on host-biomaterials and microbial interactions. Dent Mater 2019;35:36–52.
62. Huang B, Sadeghinejad L, Adebayo OIA, et al. Gene expression and protein synthesis of esterase from *Streptococcus mutans* are affected by biodegradation by-product from methacrylate resin composites and adhesives. Acta Biomater 2018;81:158–68.
63. do Amaral GS, Negrini T, Maltz M, et al. Restorative materials containing antimicrobial agents: is there evidence for their antimicrobial and anticaries effects? A systematic review. Aust Dent J 2016;61:6–15.
64. Cheng L, Zhang K, Zhang N, et al. Developing a new generation of antimicrobial and bioactive dental resins. J Dent Res 2017;96:855–63.
65. Pereira-Cenci T, Cenci MS, Fedorowicz Z, et al. Antibacterial agents in composite restorations for the prevention of dental caries. Cochrane Database Syst Rev 2013;(12):CD007819.
66. Dionysopoulos D, Koliniotou-Koumpia E, Helvatzoglou-Antoniades M, et al. Fluoride release and recharge abilities of contemporary fluoride-containing restorative materials and dental adhesives. Dent Mater J 2013;32:296–304.
67. Mickenautsch S, Mount G, Yengopal V. Therapeutic effect of glass-ionomers: an overview of evidence. Aust Dent J 2011;56:10–5.
68. Mickenautsch S, Yengopal V. Absence of carious lesions at margins of glass-ionomer cement and amalgam restorations: an update of systematic review evidence. BMC Res Notes 2011;4:58.
69. El-Deeb HA, Mobarak EH. Microshear bond strength of high-viscosity glass-ionomer to normal and caries-affected dentin under simulated intrapulpal pressure. Oper Dent 2018;43:665–73.
70. McComb D, Erickson RL, Maxymiw WG, et al. A clinical comparison of glass ionomer, resin-modified glass ionomer and resin composite restorations in the treatment of cervical caries in xerostomic head and neck radiation patients. Oper Dent 2002;27:430–7.
71. Hu JY, Li YQ, Smales RJ, et al. Restoration of teeth with more-viscous glass ionomer cements following radiation-induced caries. Int Dent J 2002;52:445–8.
72. Hu JY, Chen XC, Li YQ, et al. Radiation-induced root surface caries restored with glass-ionomer cement placed in conventional and ART cavity preparations: results at two years. Aust Dent J 2005;50:186–90.
73. De Moor RJ, Stassen IG, van't Veldt Y, et al. Two-year clinical performance of glass ionomer and resin composite restorations in xerostomic head- and neck-irradiated cancer patients. Clin Oral Investig 2011;15:31–8.
74. van de Sande FH, Rodolpho PA, Basso GR, et al. 18-year survival of posterior composite resin restorations with and without glass ionomer cement as base. Dent Mater 2015;31:669–75.
75. Alonso V, Darriba IL, Caserío M. Retrospective evaluation of posterior composite resin sandwich restorations with Herculite XRV: 18-year findings. Quintessence Int 2017;48:93–101.
76. Magne P, Silva S, Andrada M, et al. Fatigue resistance and crack propensity of novel "super-closed" sandwich composite resin restorations in large MOD defects. Int J Esthet Dent 2016;11:82–97.
77. Opdam NJ, Bronkhorst EM, Roeters JM, et al. Longevity and reasons for failure of sandwich and total-etch posterior composite resin restorations. J Adhes Dent 2007;9:469–75.

78. Friedl K, Hiller KA, Friedl KH. Clinical performance of a new glass ionomer based restoration system: a retrospective cohort study. Dent Mater 2011;27:1031–7.
79. Mickenautsch S, Yengopal V. Failure rate of direct high-viscosity glass-ionomer versus hybrid resin composite restorations in posterior permanent teeth—a systematic review. Open Dent J 2015;9:438–48.
80. Soares LE, Soares AL, De Oliveira R, et al. The effects of acid erosion and remineralization on enamel and three different dental materials: FT-Raman spectroscopy and scanning electron microscopy analysis. Microsc Res Tech 2016;79: 646–56.
81. Braga RR. Calcium phosphates as ion-releasing fillers in restorative resin-based materials. Dent Mater 2019;35:3–14.
82. Rajasekharan S, Martens LC, Cauwels RG, et al. Biodentine™ material characteristics and clinical applications: a 3 year literature review and update. Eur Arch Paediatr Dent 2018;19:1–22.
83. Kaup M, Dammann CH, Schäfer E, et al. Shear bond strength of Biodentine, Pro-Root MTA, glass ionomer cement and composite resin on human dentine ex vivo. Head Face Med 2015;11:14.
84. Butt N, Talwar S, Chaudhry S, et al. Comparison of physical and mechanical properties of mineral trioxide aggregate and Biodentine. Indian J Dent Res 2014;25:692–7.
85. Hashem D, Mannocci F, Patel S, et al. Clinical and radiographic assessment of the efficacy of calcium silicate indirect pulp capping: a randomized controlled clinical trial. J Dent Res 2015;94:562–8.
86. Hashem D, Mannocci F, Patel S, et al. Evaluation of the efficacy of calcium silicate vs. glass ionomer cement indirect pulp capping and restoration assessment criteria: a randomised controlled clinical trial-2-year results. Clin Oral Investig 2019;23(4):1931–9.
87. Koubi G, Colon P, Franquin JC, et al. Clinical evaluation of the performance and safety of a new dentine substitute, Biodentine, in the restoration of posterior teeth—a prospective study. Clin Oral Investig 2013;17:243–9.
88. Demarco FF, Corrêa MB, Cenci MS, et al. Longevity of posterior composite restorations: not only a matter of materials. Dent Mater 2012;28:87–101.
89. Collares K, Opdam NJ, Peres KG, et al. Higher experience of caries and lower income trajectory influence the quality of restorations: a multilevel analysis in a birth cohort. J Dent 2018;68:79–84.
90. Vallittu PK, Boccaccini AR, Hupa L, et al. Bioactive dental materials—do they exist and what does bioactivity mean? Dent Mater 2018;34:693–4.
91. van Dijken JWV, Pallesen U, Benetti A. A randomized controlled evaluation of posterior resin restorations of an altered resin modified glass-ionomer cement with claimed bioactivity. Dent Mater 2019;35:335–43.

Third-Party Perspective of Dental Caries Management

Frederick Eichmiller, DDS

KEYWORDS

- Insurance • Payer • Dental benefits • Reimbursement • Payment reform
- Value-based payment

KEY POINTS

- The existing fee-for-service model of reimbursement is counterproductive to the intent and delivery of caries management.
- Changing the model of reimbursement requires addressing the needs and concerns of all the stakeholders involved in making dental benefit decisions, the delivery of care, and payment for that care.
- Any new model must allocate payment based on value as perceived by the patient, and value is defined as outcomes per total dollar spent during the full cycle of care.
- A hierarchical model of outcomes measures could be used to establish the patient-centric value of dental caries management and to administer a reformed reimbursement system.
- Dental caries management could provide a unique and early opportunity to test pilot models of reformed reimbursement.

It is safe to say that every payer in today's health care market would prefer to be reimbursing for health outcomes over the current procedure-based payment system. The current fee-for-service system impedes models of care, such as caries management, by rewarding treatment over prevention, and proportionally rewarding more complex or intensive treatment over less invasive approaches to disease management. If one were to objectively assess this set of counterincentives you would have to ask how we got here and how we can ever break this counterproductive cycle. To make real and meaningful change we need to understand why and how we got here. We also need to understand and acknowledge the constraints of the current system and how many of these constraints will impact any type of proposed reform.

The first reality is that the current fee-for-service system is ingrained in our long history, tradition, and business model of dental care. Almost our entire delivery system is based on this model and we know and understand little else. We also know it is

Disclosure Statement: Delta Dental of Wisconsin is an administrator of dental benefits for employer-sponsored and individual plans.
Delta Dental of Wisconsin, 2801 Hoover Road, Stevens Point, WI 54481, USA
E-mail address: feichmiller@deltadentalwi.com

Dent Clin N Am 63 (2019) 731–736
https://doi.org/10.1016/j.cden.2019.05.005
dental.theclinics.com

inherently flawed, but we have yet to put forward an acceptable and workable alternative. The flaws become even more apparent when considering the application of this system to caries management. The basis of caries management is to reduce the morbidity and progression of disease, goals that inherently reduce the future intensity of restorative services and resulting financial rewards.[1,2] Our entire system is based on rewarding for doing more over doing less or doing better. Reforming this system, however, requires more than simply changing the way we reimburse providers. Our system of payment must also be acceptable and understandable to everyone that contributes toward that reimbursement. This includes patients; employers; governments; third-party payers; and all of the agents, brokers, consultants, and human resource administrators that play a role in the current payment systems. Consumers are also pushing for much greater transparency in payment systems, so any reform needs to be comprehensible, accessible, and highly transparent.

The second reality is that in any system there are only so many dollars available and health care economics are all about the allocation of those dollars. As a profession, dentistry has always valued prevention, but not to the degree that it places economic value on restoration and rehabilitation. Claims data show that more than 70% of procedures delivered in a dental office are diagnostic and preventive, yet these two categories make up less than 40% of the office revenue.[3] The approximately 15% of procedures dedicated to restorative generates more than 30% of revenue. Applying caries management to this scenario will only further distort this misbalance of allocation as the intensity of preventive and diagnostics increases and restorative needs decrease. Reform that supports caries management will need to either change this system of economic allocation or do away with procedure-based allocation entirely.

The third consideration is resistance to change. Every industry grapples with change management and caries management is a change that impacts every stakeholder involved in the episode of care. Providers have to accept that restoration may not be the best and first option, that tooth damage and disease are not synonymous, and that the value associated with controlling this disease must be viewed through the eyes of the patient. These are difficult concepts for a profession that has been trained that caries removal is a cure, that technical excellence in a restoration defines quality, and that monitoring and managing ongoing disease could be considered professional neglect. We have been trained to fix things and not manage or limit the damage. But resistance to change goes far beyond simply providers. Employers and sponsors that pay for care are also resistant to change. They want dental benefits to be "low noise," easy to explain, and low maintenance. They want to know their return-on-investment for any benefit reallocation or change in benefits. It is also hard to influence this perspective when dental is such a small part of their total health care spend. The same thing could be said for government programs, where dental makes up just a few percent of the total spend. Consumers also exhibit some of the same behaviors. Many payers have tested the market with innovative plan designs tailored to retirees and the individual markets, only to find that consumers desire the comfort of having a plan "just like the one I had at work." A review of available individual dental plans reveals that they still tend to follow the same general benefit designs as employer-based plans.[4–6] Another consideration related to change is the impact of the dental business model. Small independent businesses cannot afford to assume the risks associated with overhauling a payment model. An error or miscalculation in that model could put them in an unsustainable position. It is easy to see why they would resist broad-scale reform. That entrepreneurial business model, however, is also changing with larger and larger entities becoming part of the dental delivery marketplace. These larger provider organizations are testing reformed models of reimbursement, because they are better able to spread that risk across their entire business enterprise. Change is hard, but everything changes. As we try to implement a disease management approach to caries we need to keep in mind that it is not just about changing provider behavior, but rather about changing the behavior and expectations of everyone connected to delivering that model.

There are numerous books and programs outlining how to manage change within organizations, but one thing that is central to all approaches is communication. To be successful we need to clearly communicate and educate all of the relevant stakeholders on what caries management is; why it is important; the improvement that it can make in outcomes; and how it can be integrated into the delivery systems, benefit systems, and the daily lives of consumers of care. Every stakeholder will go through similar stages of denial, resistance, exploration, and acceptance. We need to be prepared for and have the tools and information to help each stakeholder work through these stages. An insurance benefits advisor may need to know how caries management can reduce client costs, an employer may be interested in how it might impact employee absenteeism, a wellness vendor may want to see the impact on comorbidities, a provider needs to know the impact on office resources and income, and government plan administrators may focus on the impact to access. Every stakeholder in the process of delivering and paying for caries management needs to be on-board to facilitate the total system of change.

Because we currently do not have any real world examples of a value-based approach to reimbursing caries management, we can still formulate a "thought experiment," or "Gedankenexperiment" to explore the possibilities. If we were to put together a thought experiment, or a payer's Gedankenexperiment around a totally new approach to reimbursing caries management, what might that look like? The first and most overriding element would be the need to sell every stakeholder on the value of the program. In health care we hear a lot about cost, quality, safety, and patient experience, but rarely do we hear about value. Porter[7] pointed out that the different stakeholders in health care often have different and often conflicting goals, but the one overarching goal common among all of them should be achieving value for patients. Value in health care can most simply be defined as outcomes relative to costs. If the goal is patient value, then everything going into the determination of value needs to be defined from the perspective of the patient. The outcomes that we measure need to be relevant to the patient and based on the perception of the patient rather than our own interpretation of intrinsic value. Such outcomes as patient comfort, speed to recovery, sustainability of health, and elimination of adverse reactions are all examples of health outcomes that directly translate to patient perceived value.

Value also needs to be measured over a full cycle or episode of care. Counting procedures and measuring processes may lead to internal process improvement, but rarely can this capture a full cycle of all the services and activities connected to comprehensive patient care. An example in caries management is that counting fluoride or silver diamine fluoride treatments might provide information that could lead to higher use of prevention, but would ignore all of the collateral services, such as nutritional counseling, home-care adjuncts, case management, and education, that are integral parts of the full cycle of caries management. Better yet, what if we measured the impact of all of these services on disease progression, normal tooth eruption, reduction in treatment needs, or reduction in lost school or work days?

Outcomes also need to be measured over longer periods. Health circumstances, such as retention of primary teeth, normal tooth eruption, and need for tooth replacement, are long-term health consequences impacted by caries management. We need to look at the outcomes from the immediate cycle of care and also the consequences of that care later on in life to establish true value. Conserving a primary dentition is a laudable goal, but has much less value if it does not lead to a healthy, functioning, permanent dentition.

If patient-centered outcomes are the numerator of value, what makes up the denominator? The cost denominator should include all of the associated costs of care for the entire care cycle. This includes not just the benefit payer's costs, but also employer contributions and patient out-of-pocket. In an ideal setting it would also include the costs of associated comorbidities, lost work place productivity, transportation, child care, and many of the hidden costs we do not normally tie into direct health care costs.

To put our hypothetical case together, let us try to apply Porter's three-tiered system of outcome measure hierarchy to caries management.[8] In Porter's hierarchy, tier 1 is the measure of health status achieved or retained over the cycle of care. The first level in that tier is survival. Fortunately, mortality from dental caries measured over any time period is low, but not zero. We all recall the tragic story of Demonte Driver[9] and each year there are deaths tied to the treatment of caries or complications related directly to the disease. One paper describing 44 cases of child deaths reported in the general media from 1980 to 2011 found that 32 of those cases were related to restorative or tooth extraction procedures and 30 were associated with moderate sedation or general anesthesia.[10] Although deaths related to dental treatment may be rare, it is still one outcome that can and, unfortunately, does occur.

The second level in tier 1 is degree of health recovery. This is measured when the patient is considered to be at a steady state achieved after completing an entire cycle of care. Outcomes related to the degree of recovery in dental caries management could include elimination of pain and infection, patient-rated function and aesthetics, new caries rates, and number of retained teeth. These are outcomes that impact the patient's sense of well-being and are of importance to how a patient would value the success of the care cycle. Tools, such as dental quality-of-life assessments, can capture the patient's perception of recovery success, whereas direct measures of biologic markers, such as tooth loss, infections, and new disease, provide objective measures of recovery. Other potential markers of recovery that could be considered are lost work/school days, emergency dental treatment, dentally related emergency department use, or hospitalizations.

Tier 2 in Porter's hierarchy is made up of measures that reflect the process of recovery. The first level in this tier is the time required to achieve recovery or return to normal function. Again, from a patient's perspective the shortest time to complete a treatment plan, the time to eliminate discomfort or regain complete function, and the number of visits necessary to complete the cycle of care would all be valid measures within this level. Level two in this tier is comprised of measures that reflect the disutility of the care or treatment process. This could include measures of patient discomfort during and after treatment; retreatment needs; failed treatments resulting in tooth loss or pulpal therapy; post-treatment complications, such as extraction site infections; and short-term restoration replacements. These are all measures of added morbidity that are associated with the treatment delivered, and not necessarily the disease state driving the additional treatment needs. These types of measures could play a large role in affirming the greater value of caries management, where more invasive treatment options could carry a higher risk for complications and adverse outcomes.

Tier 3 is comprised of measures reflecting the sustainability of health recovery. From the patient perspective the value of achieving a successful outcome matters most if that outcome can be maintained over time. The first level in this tier relates to recurrence of disease or longer-term complications of the disease. Recurrent or new caries would be one measure. Normal retention and exfoliation of primary teeth for children and retention of functional teeth in adults would be others. Longer-term retreatment needs or the needs for more complex or invasive treatment, such as root canals and crowns, fall into this level. Quality of life assessments can also provide a patient perspective of how they rate the success of their care. The second level in the health recovery tier includes the long-term consequences of care. Every intervention has long-term consequences and this level attempts to define some measure of those consequences. For caries management that may be orthodontic needs stemming from early tooth loss, tooth replacement needs for permanent tooth loss, persistent or recurrent pain, or temporomandibular joint problems associated with occlusal disharmony.

Einstein was able to translate his theory of general relativity via his Gendankenexperiment, so how do we translate this thought model of value-based reimbursement to caries management? First, we need to communicate the value of caries management clearly and concisely to all the parties involved in this cycle of care. Focusing on providers, patients, and even policy makers is not enough. The value must be understood by everyone participating in the benefit decision process, and everyone contributing to the delivery of and payment for care. Next we need to develop measures based on outcomes rather than processes. There are no shortage of potential measures, but we need to put our own value systems aside and look at outcomes purely from the perspective of patients. We could start with just a few examples from Porter's three tiers of hierarchy. One could envision a system with a base capitation rate and an allocation earned via the outcome measures. Capitation would need to be risk and disease stratified to account for the large variation in initial disease state among individuals and populations. The disease burden, management needs, and challenges in care are much different for children versus older adults, and much different for subsets within those populations. Payment systems need to reflect these differences in the capitation and earned value payments. In a successful caries management world the stratification should decline over time as patient populations benefit from the longer cycle of care. The value-based payment would need to also reward this population improvement in disease and risk stratification. This system would reward the outcomes earned from effective caries prevention and management rather than cost-shift payment to restorations.

No existing delivery or payment system can afford to take the risk of making sweeping, system-wide changes to an economic model. Change will likely come in smaller pilot programs, where risk is managed by the larger system and where greater agility is applied to modifying and improving approaches. Caries management may provide an excellent opportunity to test these pilot programs. We have well-defined populations of need in high-risk children and older adult populations. The tools for prevention and management are well tested and available, and there has been good progress in developing the risk and disease assessment methods to stratify or risk-adjust those populations. What we lack most are the outcomes measures to administer the effective allocation of value-based payments. There are some early models currently being tested, but they rely primarily on process measures and not true outcomes.[11–13]

Thought experiments are intriguing, but only have value when translated into reality. To build a value-based payment system around caries management we need to concentrate a great deal of our efforts into two areas: communication and outcomes measurement. The dental community needs to effectively communicate the patient-centered value of caries management in a way that appeals to all the players involved in benefit decisions, care delivery, and payment. At the same time, payers and providers need to build a hierarchical model of outcome-based measures that allocates payment based on providing and measuring greater value through caries management. From a payer's perspective caries management would provide an excellent model to test value-based payment. With the current emphasis on changing how we reimburse health care in medicine, this is certain to occur for dental. Caries management may be the best opportunity to begin reshaping our future.

REFERENCES

1. Evans RW, Clark P, Jia N. The caries management system: are preventive effects sustained post clinical trial? Community Dent Oral Epidemiol 2016;44(2):188–97.
2. Warren E, Curtis BH, Jia N, et al. The caries management system: updating cost-effectiveness with 4-year post trial data. Int J Technol Assess Health Care 2016; 32(3):107–15.
3. Eichmiller FC. Delta Dental of Wisconsin internal book of business claims data, CY2017. Delta Dental of Wisconsin data warehouse.
4. Delta dental individual and family plans. Available at: https://www.deltadentalcoversme.com/s/plans-by-state. Accessed April 16, 2019.
5. Humana dental insurance. Available at: https://www.humana.com/dental-insurance. Accessed April 16, 2019.
6. eHealth affordable dental insurance. Available at: https://www.ehealthinsurance.com/dental-insurance. Accessed April 16, 2019.
7. Institute of Medicine. Evidence-based medicine and the changing nature of health care: 2007 IOM annual meeting summary. In: Porter ME, editor. Defining and introducing value in health care. Washington, DC: The National Academies Press; 2008. p. 161–72.
8. Porter ME. What is value in health care? N Engl J Med 2010;363(26):2477–81.
9. Otto M. For want of a dentist. Washington Post, Wednesday, February 28, 2007. Available at: http://www.washingtonpost.com/wp-dyn/content/article/2007/02/27/AR2007022702116.html?noredirect=on. Accessed April 16, 2019.
10. Lee HH, Milgrom P, Starks H, et al. Trends in death associated with pediatric dental sedation and general anesthesia. Paediatr Anaesth 2013;23(8):741–6.
11. Centers for Medicare & Medicaid Services. Medicaid innovation accelerator program: children's oral health care delivery models and value-based payment approaches: key findings from an environmental scan 2018. Available at: https://www.medicaid.gov/state-resource-center/innovation-accelerator-program/iap-functional-areas/value-based-payment/index.html. Accessed April 16, 2019.
12. Oregon Health Authority. Oregon health system transformation: CCO metrics 2017 final report 2018. Available at: https://www.oregon.gov/oha/HPA/ANALYTICS/Pages/index.aspx. Accessed April 16, 2019.
13. Massachusetts Executive Office of Health and Human Services. MCO administered ACO model contract, appendix B: EOHHS accountable care organization quality appendix 2017. Available at: https://www.mass.gov/lists/mco-administered-aco-model-contract-and-model-appendices. Accessed April 16, 2019.

Less Is More? The Long-Term Health and Cost Consequences Resulting from Minimal Invasive Caries Management

Falk Schwendicke, PhD, MDPH

KEYWORDS

- Caries • Costs • Decision making • Economics • Effectiveness • Modeling • Trials

KEY POINTS

- Caries management is a long-term exercise, and comprehensive and applicable health economic analyses on caries management strategies should accordingly attempt to use a long-term perspective.
- A range of factors, such as an individual's caries risk, the tooth or lesion to be treated, the setting and the study methodology, affect the outcomes of health economic studies.
- Researchers should record data on costs in their studies. Patients and dentists should be aware of the interplay between effectiveness and costs.
- Health economic analyses are useful to support decision making in health services organization and commissioning.
- Minimal invasive caries management is often, but not always, more effective, but also less costly, especially in the long term.

INTRODUCTION

Dental caries is a chronic, behaviorally determined, and bacterially associated disease. Considering that teeth are present from early life onward, and especially in a patient with risky behavior (frequent carbohydrate consumption, poor oral hygiene, limited supply of topical fluorides), teeth are at risk of developing carious lesions from early in their life, with long-term sequelae.[1–3] Any management strategy for dental caries has both initial and long-term consequences; these involve the preservation or generation of health (or the occurrence of adverse events) as well as the costs generated. This article discusses the long-term health and costs consequences resulting from different caries management strategies.

Disclosure: The author has nothing to disclose.
Department for Operative and Preventive Dentistry, Charité – Universitätsmedizin Berlin, Aßmannshauser Str. 4-6, Berlin 14197, Germany
E-mail address: falk.schwendicke@charite.de

Dent Clin N Am 63 (2019) 737–749
https://doi.org/10.1016/j.cden.2019.06.006
0011-8532/19/© 2019 Elsevier Inc. All rights reserved.

dental.theclinics.com

HEALTH AND COSTS ARE ASSOCIATED

Most caries management strategies are not a permanent "fix" for dental caries, because it will require repetition or some kind of re-treatment in the future. For example, the preventive application of fluoride varnish usually requires repetition, and not all lesions will be prevented; hence, even surfaces that had received a fluoride varnish some years previously may develop a carious lesion, and this lesion could progress to a status where a restoration is needed. Also, a restoration seldom lasts a lifetime, but rather fails after a statistically defined period—which may be 5 or 25 years depending on the restoration material, the operator, and, first and foremost, the patient. Similarly, a re-intervention on a restoration may involve a repair or a replacement, again with chances that further treatments may be needed. The cycle of long-term interventions resulting from dental caries has been termed the "cycle of re-interventions," "restorative cycle," or "death spiral of restorations," with all terms emphasizing that restorative interventions are not unlimitedly repeatable: each re-restoration is larger than the previous one and, at some stage, dentists may run out of restorative options, requiring the tooth to be removed (**Fig. 1**). In short, caries management is a lifetime story.[4–6]

Any caries management strategy will thus either preserve health (eg, avoiding the occurrence of carious lesions), regain health (by restoring cavities and tooth functionality or esthetics), or lose health (if a treatment fails, for example if the pulp is exposed in a carious tooth during operative interventions). Regardless of this health gain or loss, each procedure incurs costs. However, not only the initial caries management, but also the described re-treatment of caries and carious lesions generates costs. These costs may be lower, as high as, or often even higher than the initial costs; the latter mainly because re-treatments will often be more extensive and complex (eg, repeated re-restoration of a tooth, for example, may eventually involve crowns; tooth

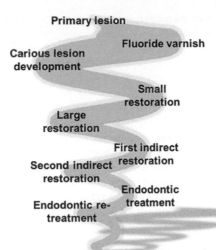

Fig. 1. Spiral of re-interventions, also termed "death spiral of the tooth" or "restorative cycle." (*Data from* Qvist V. Longevity of restorations: the 'death spiral'. In: Fejerskov O, Kidd EAM, eds. *Dental Caries: The Disease and Its Clinical Management.* Vol 2. Oxford: Blackwell Munksgaard; 2008:444-455; and Brantley C, Bader J, Shugars D, Nesbit S. Does the cycle of rerestoration lead to larger restorations? *The Journal of the American Dental Association.* 1995;126(10):1407-1413.)

removal of teeth that are nonrestorable may lead to the need for a fixed or removable dental prosthesis placement or an implant-supported single crown). Hence, the initial health gains provided by an intervention will be linked to the long-term costs; saving money early on might be less relevant than being effective long term, as this may reduce long-term costs.

In summary, caries management has long-term health and costs implications. The long-term consequences of any kind of management (be it minimally invasive or not) need a long-term perspective.

METHODS FOR ASSESSING HEALTH AND COST CONSEQUENCES IN THE LONG TERM

To assess the health and cost consequences of health care in the long term, health economic analyses are usually required. Health economics distinguishes between 4 different types of analyses; these are categorized according to the measured health outcome[7]:

- Cost-cost studies. In these analyses, no health benefit is assessed, but only the costs of interventions, assuming that their effectiveness is the same (this, however, is seldom the case). The costs considered by such analyses (and generally, all health economic analyses) differ according to the perspective of the study: sometimes, only costs covered by the patient or the health care system are included, while many studies aim to consider the wider (so-called societal) costs. A range of costs can be discriminated: (1) direct medical costs (for example for diagnostics and treatment, staff, materials, drugs), (2) direct nonmedical costs (for example for patient's traveling to and from the dentist, for transportation costs between the laboratory and the dentists), (3) indirect costs (those for lost opportunities, as explained below), and (4) intangible costs (which cannot easily be quantified, eg, for stress or pain during treatment or side-effects of a medication). Indirect (often called opportunity) costs are costs generated by spending time on medical treatment (eg, attending a dentist) instead of laboring or leisuring (so-called absenteeism, ie, being absent from work), or being of lower productivity at work or enjoying leisure time to a lesser degree because of a disease (so-called presenteeism, because one is present but not fully "there"). Absenteeism includes the assessment of traveling, waiting, and treatment times, and so-forth.[8,9] Absenteeism and presenteeism times can be multiplied with a value assigned to this time (assigning these values, however, is not easy, and may be highly dependent on the individual's occupational status, or the value an individual places on his/her leisure time), resulting in a monetary value. Although cost-cost studies are rare, the described considerations around costs are relevant for all health economic analyses.
- Cost-effectiveness studies. These assess the effectiveness of a treatment (with effectiveness being defined as a clinically measurable outcome, such as avoided DMFT [decayed, missing, and filled teeth] increment), and weigh this effectiveness against the costs. One main outcome parameter of these studies is the incremental cost-effectiveness ratio (ICER), which is the cost-difference of 2 interventions divided by the effectiveness difference. The ICER is usually a positive value and indicates the additional money a decision maker needs to spend to buy an increment of better health, assuming that the better treatment is more expensive, which is often the case. Sometimes, however, a more expensive treatment is less effective, or a less expensive one is also more effective; in these cases, the ICER is negative, indicating that there is no decision problem.[10]
- Cost-utility studies. These investigate the utility of a treatment, which is oftentimes measured as quality-adjusted or disability-adjusted life years. To elicit

the subjective value individuals place on certain health states (like a retained tooth or an untreated carious lesion causing pain), many tools, often questionnaires, are used. Notably, the elicited values differ between settings, but also change over time, and have not been estimated for all dental health states (it is also highly complex to measure the utility value placed on 1 specific tooth and not the whole dentition). As long as utility values of different health states and organs/organ functions are elicited using the same or very similar tools (questionnaires), this also allows to compare interventions across different medical disciplines. Such analyses are useful for resource allocation.

- Cost-benefit studies. These transform effectiveness or utility, that is the health outcome, into a monetary value. This again means that interventions for various diseases and across disciplines (dentistry, rheumatology, ophthalmology) can be measured on the same scale. More importantly, health gains and costs are also identically scaled, and interpreting the health gain by money spent is easier (interpreting the effectiveness gain, such as a prevented carious lesions, per money spent is less straightforward). These analyses have only been sparsely applied in dentistry so far.

Measuring health gains and costs and the resulting cost-effectiveness/utility/benefit can be performed in 2 ways:

- The first involves collecting original data for the purpose of health economic analyses, for example, as part of a clinical (interventional or observational) study. Such data collection allows recording in detail the direct medical costs (staff hours, medical equipment used, materials consumed), direct nonmedical costs (transport costs, for example, for visiting the dental office) and indirect ones (recording traveling, waiting, and treatment times, for example). Moreover, the cost estimation and the effectiveness data collection are performed in the same setting. Alternative methods for measuring health and costs often need to use and combine data from different sources and settings (eg, university clinics, practices, even countries), as discussed below.
- The second uses mathematical models. These are built on data not necessarily collected for the purpose of a health economic evaluation, for example, on meta-analyses of various effectiveness trials, or cost estimates yielded from other studies. These data are then used to populate the model. The mathematical models used are designed to follow individuals or teeth over a defined period of time (in line with the remarks above, ideally long term, to capture the long-term cost and effectiveness consequences). Individuals or teeth "start" the modeling period in a certain health state (for example a sound surface, which is either sealed or not sealed) and can move from there to another health state (eg, to an early carious lesion) or remain in the initial health state. If they moved to the next health state, they again have the option to move further forward (to a cavitated carious lesion, for example). Modeling studies hence allow longer sequences of events (eg, sealed sound tooth → lost sealant and carious surface → restoration → replaced restoration → extracted tooth → implant). The probability of each transition between health states is based on underlying data, and each transition comes with health losses or gains, and costs (for treatment, or indirect costs for presenteeism or absenteeism, for example). Modeling has the advantage of (1) being able to consider wider evidence than a single study (using data from a meta-analysis may be more robust than data from a single study); (2) extrapolate early events long term, something which is limited in most clinical studies (clinical studies are seldom able to follow individuals over

a lifetime), (3) compare a large range of options for their costs and effectiveness (clinical studies will only compare few interventions against each other due resource constrains). However, modeling studies require a number of assumptions to be made, both in the construction of the model as well as the parameters used for modeling: they are subject to a range of uncertainties (the same, however, is true for clinical studies, where external and internal validity are limited to some degree and parameters are uncertain, too, as indicated for example by confidence intervals around any effectiveness estimates). The relevance of uncertainty is discussed next.

UNCERTAINTY IN HEALTH ECONOMICS

Different uncertainties are discriminated in health economics[11,12]: (1) structural uncertainty in the case of modeling studies (the structure of the model may affect the study outcome and should be varied to gauge the impact of the model structure on study findings); (2) heterogeneity (interventions in patients with different age or risk or profile, anterior or posterior teeth, proximal and occlusal surfaces all come with a possible different cost and effectiveness profile); and (3) parameter uncertainty (any parameter, be it the effectiveness estimate of a single study or a meta-analysis, as well as most cost input parameters, are not 100% certain).

All these uncertainties can be evaluated, for example, using univariate sensitivity analyses. Such analyses may vary an aspect of the study, for example, a structural component of the model, a patient's caries risk profile, or an input parameter (such as the costs for the application of a fluoride varnish by a dental nurse instead of a dentist) to explore the importance of the uncertainty for the study findings. Obviously, modeling studies allow variation of a far greater number of parameters than clinical studies (clinical studies need to include different subgroups, for example, to evaluate the relevance of heterogeneity). Alternatively, modeling studies may vary all uncertain parameters jointly, which allows to quantify the overall uncertainty of a study outcome.

Uncertainty analyses are most relevant to inform decision makers. Consider, for example, a study comparing the costs and effectiveness of different interventions. If the ranking of interventions remains unchanged despite large uncertainty, this uncertainty may be acceptable for decision makers. In contrast, if an only small uncertainty in a study will nevertheless reverse the ranking of interventions, decision makers may not make a decision based on information gained by this study as it is too ambiguous.

THE COST-EFFECTIVENESS OF MINIMAL INVASIVE CARIES MANAGEMENT

In the following sections, the cost-effectiveness of different caries management strategies is discussed. First, caries prevention using fluoride varnish in children is discussed. Subsequently, the cost-effectiveness of different carious tissue removal strategies, as well as the Hall Technique, are presented. Finally, the cost-effectiveness of restoration renewal versus repair for partially defective restorations is discussed.

Cost-Effectiveness of Caries Prevention Using Fluoride Varnish

Professionally applied fluoride varnishes are known to be effective to reduce caries increment.[13,14] However, varnish application generates costs (for the material and the staff who apply it, but also indirect costs as described above for patients attending the dentist). These initial costs for the application of the varnish may be compensated long term, if caries increment and the subsequent need for (relatively expensive) retreatments (mainly restorations) can be avoided. There is a larger number of studies assessing the cost-effectiveness of fluoride varnish application; most of them, however, did not take a long-term perspective.[15-18] A recent study[19] used a simulation model to follow teeth which received in-office application of fluoride varnish versus those which did not over the lifetime of initially 12-year-old individuals. The study took a mixed public-private-payer perspective in Germany, where most of the population is covered by (statutory) public insurance, which covers nearly all (except very advanced or prosthetic) treatments. Treatments which are not covered are paid privately or by an additional private insurer (hence mixed perspective).[20] To assess the impact of different caries risk, 3 risk groups (low, medium, and high risk) were additionally discriminated during modeling. A biannual application of fluoride varnish until age 18 was compared with no fluoride application. The effectiveness of the varnish application was derived from systematic reviews. The health outcome was caries increment (DMFT). Cost calculations were based on the fees German dentists would claim from the insurance and/or the individual; these fees are fixed and recorded in fee item catalogs.[21] Future costs and effectiveness were discounted at 3% per annum.[22] Discounting accounts for the fact that individuals value opportunities lost (money spent, health lost) or gained (money saved, health gained) now more highly than opportunities lost or gained in the future.

Initially, the individual was assumed to have 28 sound teeth. Depending on his or her caries risk, teeth had a certain probability of carious lesion development. This risk was modified (decreased) when fluoride varnish was assumed to be applied.[13,14] If a carious lesion occurred (ie, caries increment), this was assumed to result in the placement of an adhesive composite restoration. If this restoration failed, re-restoration using another composite or further restorative strategies was modeled. Also, endodontic complications (leading to nonsurgical primary or secondary root-canal treatment or surgical re-treatment, ie, apicectomy, or extraction) were considered. If teeth needed extraction, tooth replacement via implant-supported crowns was simulated. Implants and implant-supported crowns were assumed to be prone to restorative complications (requiring re-cementation or renewal of crowns) as well as biologic (eg, peri-implantitis with subsequent implant loss) or technical complications (like abutment or implant fracture) according to a range of data sources. In short, the model aimed to simulate the whole restorative spiral shown in **Fig. 1**.

The initial costs for the varnish were assumed to range between 12 and 14 Euro per application. Over the patients' lifetime and as a mean of all risk groups, not applying fluoride during age 12 to 18 was the least costly (230 Euro), but also the least effective, strategy (mean caries increment was 11 DMFT). Applying the varnish was more costly, but also more effective (357 Euro, DMFT 7). The ICER was 39 Euro per avoided DMFT when the varnish was applied. The so-called cost-effectiveness plane is shown in **Fig. 2**.

In high-risk patients, costs for both strategies (no fluoride varnish, 389 Euro; fluoride varnish, 515 Euro) were higher, and effectiveness lower (13 and 10 DMFT), leading to an identical ICER of 39 Euro. In contrast, in low-risk individuals, the costs were much lower (24 and 174 Euro), and the effectiveness higher (2 and 1 DMFT). The ICER, notably, was much higher, at 193 Euro/DMFT. The study concluded that in-office fluoride application was likely more effective, but also more costly, than no fluoride application, especially in low-risk individuals. A general aspect emerging from this study was that caries prevention does not necessarily save costs. Cost savings will depend on the relative and absolute effectiveness of such an application, but also initial and follow-up treatment costs. For example, had a nurse applied the fluoride varnish (maybe even out of office, eg, in a school), initial (and total) costs may have been lower. If fluoride varnish had a higher relative effectiveness, the cost-effectiveness of the varnish would have been higher.

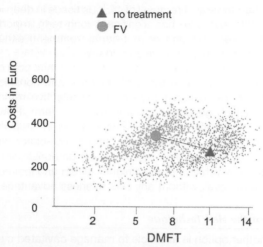

Fig. 2. Cost-effectiveness plane of fluoride varnish (FV) application and of no such applica-tion.[19] The mean costs and DMFT values of bootstrapped modeled populations are shown. The large quadrangle and triangle indicate the overall mean of all samples. FV was more costly but also more effective than no treatment. (*Data from* Schwendicke F, Stolpe M. In-Office Application of Fluoride Gel or Varnish: Cost-Effectiveness and Expected Value of Perfect Information Analysis. *Caries Res.* 2017;51(3):231-239.)

Cost-Effectiveness of Carious Tissue Removal Strategies

In another cost-effectiveness evaluation, different carious tissue removal strategies (ie, nonselective, selective and stepwise) have been compared.[23] This is a specific case, as at least nonselective and selective removal do not have different initial costs (they come with similar treatment efforts and materials needed, at least when no spe-cific tool for selective removal is used). Stepwise removal generates higher initial costs because of a second visit, including a re-entry and re-restoration, being needed.

The study focused on the treatment of deep carious lesions, which come with sig-nificant risks for the integrity of the pulp.[24] Pulp exposure and complications often lead to a cascade of escalating re-interventions.[25] Selective or stepwise removals have been found to reduce these risks compared with nonselective removal. The study simulated the management of a molar tooth with a deep lesion in an initially 15-year-old child. Again, systematically compiled and meta-analyzed effectiveness data, allowing the comparison of the risks of pulp exposure, pulp complications, and restorative complications between the 3 removal strategies, were used to assign transition probabilities (eg, carious tissue removal → pulp exposure → direct capping → root-canal treatment → endodontic complications), allowing a lifelong follow-up of treated teeth. Again, the study adopted a mixed public-private-payer perspective within German health care, and the cost estimation was performed as described. The primary health outcome was the time teeth were retained (in years); note that such analyses are usually not possible in clinical studies (because tooth loss often happens 20, 30, or 40 years after the initial treatment). The secondary health outcome was the time pulp vitality was maintained.

Selective carious tissue removal had lower long-term costs (265 Euro), and retained teeth and pulp vitality for longer (means: 53.5 and 41.0 years) than stepwise removal (360 Euro, 52.5 and 37.5 years) and nonselective removal (398 Euro, 49.5 and 31.0 years). This analysis confirmed the relevance of the long-term consequences resulting from the initial strategy of removal of carious tissue in deep lesions for overall cost-effectiveness. Pulp exposure has significant long-term importance, mainly as follow-up treatments (direct capping or root-canal-treatment) either have relatively poor success rates or are rather invasive and costly.

Stepwise removal, notably, was initially more expensive than both other options, but its long-term costs ranged between those of selective and nonselective removal. It compensated its initial cost-disadvantage over nonselective removal by requiring fewer re-treatments (which generate costs) in the long term. However, compared with selective removal, its effectiveness remained lower; stepwise removal was more costly and less effective. This disadvantageous cost-effectiveness of stepwise compared with selective removal has recently been demonstrated by a short-term study in primary molars, which found much higher (direct and indirect) costs for stepwise versus selective removal, without any effectiveness advantage.[26]

Cost-Effectiveness of the Hall Technique

In primary teeth, another option is available to manage cavitated carious lesions; the Hall Technique, in which carious tissue is sealed beneath stainless steel crowns.[27] Hall Technique has been discussed in this series of articles, and a range of studies also assessed its cost-effectiveness.[28–30] These studies, notably, used different designs (both a model and original data were used for analyses) and were conducted in different settings (the United Kingdom and Germany). All studies agreed that the Hall Technique was more expensive initially than the comparators, notably nonselective removal followed by conventional direct restorations and (in 1 German study) nonrestorative cavity control (NRCC). Also, all studies reported the Hall Technique to be more effective in reducing both pulp and restorative complications. In 2 of these studies,[28,29] indirect costs were also quantified, which makes a difference when considering that for NRCC, for example, repeated visits in short intervals are needed. Also, repeated restoration failure (as is the case for many direct restorations in primary dentition) comes with high indirect costs.

In all 3 studies, the Hall Technique had a significantly higher cost-effectiveness than alternatives, regardless of its higher initial costs. These analyses on the cost-effectiveness of the Hall Technique are a good example of robust information; the 3 studies were performed in different settings and on different populations, with different perspectives and horizons, and used different analytical methods, but came to the same conclusion based on similar findings (**Fig. 3**).

Cost-Effectiveness of Restoration Repair

Treatment of failed restorations is the most frequently performed dental activity in many countries; up to 60% of all treatments performed by general dentists are restoration re-treatments.[31–35] Traditionally, a partially defective restoration was completely removed under the assumption that this would be needed for the re-treatment to be long-lasting. However, as described elsewhere in this series of articles, repairing partially defective restorations (eg, including also resealing, repolishing) has become more accepted, because it avoids further (possibly unnecessary) removal of sound dental hard tissue,[36–38] which may limit the longevity of the tooth in the long term.[39–41] Also, repair restorations may save time and, hence, be, at least initially, less costly than completely replacing them.[42] However, repaired restorations may show lower survival probability (requiring more—costly—re-treatments) than completely replaced restorations,[43,44] which might compensate for possible initial cost savings.

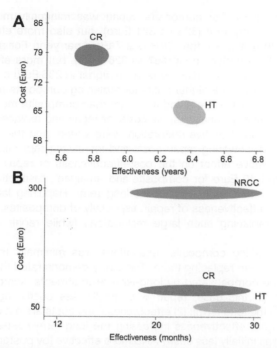

Fig. 3. Cost-effectiveness planes comparing the Hall Technique (HT) against conventional carious tissue removal and restoration (CR) or, in 1 study, nonrestorative cavity control (NRCC). Results from 2 studies, 1 using a model (*A*) and 1 using data from a randomized trial (*B*) using tooth retention years as outcome for the cost-effectiveness analysis. The 95% CIs of costs (Euro) and effectiveness (survival in years, months) of the 3 strategies (HT, Hall Technique, orange; NRCC, nonrestorative cavity control, green; CR, conventional restorative treatment, blue) are plotted as ellipses. HT was more effective (being situated at the right hand side of the plane) and less costly (being situated at the bottom of the plane) compared with other interventions. (*Data from* [*A*] Schwendicke F, Stolpe M, Innes N. Conventional treatment, Hall Technique or immediate pulpotomy for carious primary molars: a cost-effectiveness analysis. *International Endodontic Journal.* 2016;49(9):817-826; and [*B*] Schwendicke F, Krois J, Splieth CH, et al. Cost-effectiveness of managing cavitated primary molar caries lesions: A randomized trial In Germany. *Journal of Dentistry.* 2018.)

A recent study used a model to analyze restoration repair versus replacement.[45] Again, a mixed public-private-payer perspective in the context of the German health care setting was used. Sixty-year-old individuals with 1 permanent molar with a 3-surfaced partially defective composite or amalgam restorations were followed over their remaining lifetime. Again, in both strategies (repair, replace), several complications were modeled, including another restorative failure, leading to further re-restorations, endodontic complications, and extractions. The proportions of the different re-treatments were estimated based on a large, practice-based study from the Netherlands, which had followed repaired and replaced restorations in the long term.[43,46] Also, for the follow-up health states, a range of restorative complications (eg, crown de-cementation, fracture, or secondary caries) or endodontic complications were modeled. Extracted teeth were again assumed to be partially replaced using implant-supported single crowns, which also came with risks of complications as described.

The initial costs for replacing a partially defective composite restoration were estimated to amount to 160 Euro, amalgam replacement to 104 Euro, and repair restorations to 69 Euro. For composite, repair was minimally more costly than replacement in the long term (326 vs 321 Euro), but also more effective (24.7 vs 24.0 years of tooth retention), the ICER was 7 Euro per year. For amalgam, repair was more costly than replacement (467 vs 326 Euro), but more effective (24.3 vs 23.7 tooth retention years); the ICER was much higher at 235 Euro per year. This difference was grounded in the higher costs for replacing composite restorations, but also in the lower longevity of repaired amalgam than composite restorations.[43]

In a number of sensitivity analyses, the costs for repair and replacement, as well as the size of the partially defective restoration, were varied, and the impact on cost-effectiveness tested. Lowering repair costs and increasing replacement costs had, as expected, a positive effect on the cost-effectiveness of repair. If repair costs were below 67 and 40 Euro for composite and amalgam, respectively, repair was both more effective and less costly in the long term. Repairing large restorations increased the cost-effectiveness of repair, especially of composites, because of the higher costs for replacing such large restorations (while repair costs remained identical).

In summary, repairing composite restorations was minimally more costly, but also more effective than replacing them. This study demonstrated that (1) initial cost differences may be compensated by long-term re-treatments, something which we discussed above (in this case, repair was initially less costly, but re-treatments increased costs in the long term); (2) effectiveness and costs are not always unidirectionally linked (higher effectiveness increasing the long-term cost-effectiveness; in our case, repair was initially less costly AND more effective [by postponing the restorative cycle and thus stretching the restorative tooth loss spiral], but nevertheless more costly in the long term); and (3) heterogeneity had a great impact on cost-effectiveness (for example, there were large differences between repairing composites and amalgams, and repairing larger or smaller restorations).

SUMMARY

Caries management is a long-term exercise, and comprehensive and applicable health economic analyses on caries management strategies should accordingly attempt to use a long-term perspective. A range of factors, such as an individual's caries risk, the tooth or lesion to be treated, the setting, and the study methodology (model/original data, perspective, horizon) all affect the outcomes of health economic studies on caries management. Cariology researchers should record data on costs alongside any observational and/or intervention studies if applicable. Patients and dentists should be aware of the interplay between effectiveness and costs, with initial costs often being less decisive than the long-term effectiveness for the overall cost-effectiveness. Health economic analyses are useful to support decision making in organization and commissioning in health services. Minimal invasive caries management is not always more effective, but often less costly, especially in the long term.

REFERENCES

1. Marsh PD. In sickness and in health—what does the oral microbiome mean to us? An ecological perspective. Adv Dent Res 2018;29(1):60–5.
2. Marsh PD. Microbial ecology of dental plaque and its significance in health and disease. Adv Dent Res 1994;8(2):263–71.
3. Frencken JE, Innes NP, Schwendicke F. Managing carious lesions: why do we need consensus on terminology and clinical recommendations on carious tissue removal? Adv Dent Res 2016;28(2):46–8.

4. Qvist V. Longevity of restorations: the 'death spiral'. In: Fejerskov O, Kidd EAM, editors. Dental caries: the disease and its clinical management, vol. 2. Oxford (United Kingdom): Blackwell Munksgaard; 2008. p. 444–55.
5. Elderton RJ. Clinical studies concerning re-restoration of teeth. Adv Dent Res 1990;4:4–9.
6. Brantley C, Bader J, Shugars D, et al. Does the cycle of rerestoration lead to larger restorations? J Am Dent Assoc 1995;126(10):1407–13.
7. Vernazza C, Heasman P, Gaunt F, et al. How to measure the cost-effectiveness of periodontal treatments. Periodontol 2000 2012;60(1):138–46.
8. Klarenbach SW, Tonelli M, Chui B, et al. Economic evaluation of dialysis therapies. Nat Rev Nephrol 2014;10(11):644–52.
9. Durham J, Shen J, Breckons M, et al. Healthcare cost and impact of persistent orofacial pain: the DEEP study cohort. J Dent Res 2016;95(10):1147–54.
10. Drummond M, Stoddart G, Labelle R, et al. Health economics: an introduction for clinicians. Ann Intern Med 1987;107(1):88–92.
11. Briggs AH, O'Brien BJ, Blackhouse G. Thinking outside the box: recent advances in the analysis and presentation of uncertainty in cost-effectiveness studies. Annu Rev Public Health 2002;23(1):377–401.
12. Glick HA, Briggs AH, Polsky D. Quantifying stochastic uncertainty and presenting results of cost-effectiveness analyses. Expert Rev Pharmacoecon Outcomes Res 2001;1(1):25–36.
13. Marinho VC, Worthington HV, Walsh T, et al. Fluoride varnishes for preventing dental caries in children and adolescents. Cochrane Database Syst Rev 2013;(7):CD002279.
14. Marinho VC, Worthington HV, Walsh T, et al. Fluoride gels for preventing dental caries in children and adolescents. Cochrane Database Syst Rev 2015;(6):CD002280.
15. Marino R, Fajardo J, Morgan M. Cost-effectiveness models for dental caries prevention programmes among Chilean schoolchildren. Community Dent Health 2012;29(4):302–8.
16. Quinonez RB, Stearns SC, Talekar BS, et al. Simulating cost-effectiveness of fluoride varnish during well-child visits for Medicaid-enrolled children. Arch Pediatr Adolesc Med 2006;160(2):164–70.
17. Splieth CH, Flessa S. Modelling lifelong costs of caries with and without fluoride use. Eur J Oral Sci 2008;116(2):164–9.
18. Vermaire JH, van Loveren C, Brouwer WB, et al. Value for money: economic evaluation of two different caries prevention programmes compared with standard care in a randomized controlled trial. Caries Res 2014;48(3):244–53.
19. Schwendicke F, Stolpe M. In-office application of fluoride gel or varnish: cost-effectiveness and expected value of perfect information analysis. Caries Res 2017;51(3):231–9.
20. GKV-Spitzenverband. Beitragsbemessung. 2017. Available at: http://www.gkv-spitzenverband.de/presse/zahlen_und_grafiken/zahlen_und_grafiken.jsp#lightbox. Accessed May 01, 2019.
21. KZBV. Catalogue of fees [Gebührenverzeichnisse] 2017. 2017. Available at: http://www.kzbv.de/gebuehrenverzeichnisse.334.de.html. Accessed May 01, 2019.
22. IQWiG. Appraisal of recommendations by the scientific board of IQWiG regarding "Methods to assess cost-effectiveness in German Public Health Insurance" [Würdigung der Empfehlung des Wissenschaftlichen Beirats des IQWiG zur,,Methodik für die Bewertung von Verhältnissen zwischen Nutzen und Kosten im System der deutschen gesetzlichen Krankenversicherung"]. 2009. Available

at: https://www.iqwig.de/download/Wuerdigung_der_Stellungnahmen_KNB-Method enentwurf_2.0.pdf. Accessed July 18, 2013.

23. Schwendicke F, Stolpe M, Meyer-Lückel H, et al. Cost-effectiveness of one- and two-step incomplete and complete excavation. J Dent Res 2013; 92(10):880–7.

24. Schwendicke F, Dorfer CE, Paris S. Incomplete caries removal: a systematic review and meta-analysis. J Dent Res 2013;92(4):306–14.

25. Schwendicke F, Frencken JE, Bjorndal L, et al. Managing carious lesions: consensus recommendations on carious tissue removal. Adv Dent Res 2016; 28(2):58–67.

26. Elhennawy K, Finke C, Paris S, et al. Selective vs stepwise removal of deep carious lesions in primary molars: 12-months results of a randomized controlled pilot trial. J Dent 2018;77:72–7.

27. Innes NP, Evans DJ, Stirrups DR. Sealing caries in primary molars: randomized control trial, 5-year results. J Dent Res 2011;90(12):1405–10.

28. Schwendicke F, Krois J, Robertson M, et al. Cost-effectiveness of the hall technique in a randomized trial. J Dent Res 2018;98(1):61–7.

29. Schwendicke F, Krois J, Splieth CH, et al. Cost-effectiveness of managing cavitated primary molar caries lesions: a randomized trial in Germany. J Dent 2018; 78:40–5.

30. Schwendicke F, Stolpe M, Innes N. Conventional treatment, hall technique or immediate pulpotomy for carious primary molars: a cost-effectiveness analysis. Int Endod J 2016;49(9):817–26.

31. Braga SR, Vasconcelos BT, Macedo MR, et al. Reasons for placement and replacement of direct restorative materials in Brazil. Quintessence Int 2007; 38(4):e189–94.

32. Mjor IA, Dahl JE, Moorhead JE. Placement and replacement of restorations in primary teeth. Acta Odontol Scand 2002;60(1):25–8.

33. Tyas MJ. Placement and replacement of restorations by selected practitioners. Aust Dent J 2005;50(2):81–9 [quiz: 127].

34. Al Negrish AR. Reasons for placement and replacement of amalgam restorations in jordan. Int Dent J 2001;51(2):109–15.

35. Chrysanthakopoulos NA. Placement, replacement and longevity of composite resin-based restorations in permanent teeth in Greece. Int Dent J 2012;62(3): 161–6.

36. Gordan VV. Clinical evaluation of replacement of class V resin based composite restorations. J Dent 2001;29(7):485–8.

37. Gordan VV. In vitro evaluation of margins of replaced resin-based composite restorations. J Esthet Dent 2000;12(4):209–15.

38. Gordan VV, Mondragon E, Shen C. Replacement of resin-based composite: evaluation of cavity design, cavity depth, and shade matching. Quintessence Int 2002;33(4):273–8.

39. Kanzow P, Hoffmann R, Tschammler C, et al. Attitudes, practice and experience of german dentists regarding repair restorations. Clin Oral Investig 2017;21(4): 1087–93.

40. Gordan VV, Riley J 3rd, Geraldeli S, et al. The decision to repair or replace a defective restoration is affected by who placed the original restoration: findings from the National Dental PBRN. J Dent 2014;42(12):1528–34.

41. Gordan VV, Riley JL 3rd, Geraldeli S, et al. Repair or replacement of defective restorations by dentists in The Dental Practice-Based Research Network. J Am Dent Assoc 2012;143(6):593–601.

42. Blum IR, Hafiana K, Curtis A, et al. The effect of surface conditioning on the bond strength of resin composite to amalgam. J Dent 2012;40(1):15–21.
43. Opdam NJ, Bronkhorst EM, Loomans BA, et al. Longevity of repaired restorations: a practice based study. J Dent 2012;40(10):829–35.
44. Smales RJ, Hawthorne WS. Long-term survival of repaired amalgams, recemented crowns and gold castings. Oper Dent 2004;29(3):249–53.
45. Kanzow P, Wiegand A, Schwendicke F. Cost-effectiveness of repairing versus replacing composite or amalgam restorations. J Dent 2016;54:41–7.
46. Opdam NJ, Bronkhorst EM, Loomans BA, et al. 12-year survival of composite vs. amalgam restorations. J Dent Res 2010;89(10):1063–7.

UNITED STATES POSTAL SERVICE®

Statement of Ownership, Management, and Circulation (All Periodicals Publications Except Requester Publications)

1. Publication Title	2. Publication Number	3. Filing Date
DENTAL CLINICS OF NORTH AMERICA	566 – 480	9/18/2019

4. Issue Frequency	5. Number of Issues Published Annually	6. Annual Subscription Price
JAN, APR, JUL, OCT	4	$304.00

7. Complete Mailing Address of Known Office of Publication (Not printer) (Street, city, county, state, and ZIP+4®)

ELSEVIER INC.
230 Park Avenue, Suite 800
New York, NY 10169

Contact Person
STEPHEN R. BUSHING

Telephone (Include area code)
215-239-3688

8. Complete Mailing Address of Headquarters or General Business Office of Publisher (Not printer)

ELSEVIER INC.
230 Park Avenue, Suite 800
New York, NY 10169

9. Full Names and Complete Mailing Addresses of Publisher, Editor, and Managing Editor (Do not leave blank)

Publisher (Name and complete mailing address)

TAYLOR BALL, ELSEVIER INC.
1600 JOHN F KENNEDY BLVD. SUITE 1800
PHILADELPHIA, PA 19103-2899

Editor (Name and complete mailing address)

JOHN VASSALLO, ELSEVIER INC.
1600 JOHN F KENNEDY BLVD. SUITE 1800
PHILADELPHIA, PA 19103-2899

Managing Editor (Name and complete mailing address)

PATRICK MANLEY, ELSEVIER INC.
1600 JOHN F KENNEDY BLVD. SUITE 1800
PHILADELPHIA, PA 19103-2899

10. Owner (Do not leave blank. If the publication is owned by a corporation, give the name and address of the corporation immediately followed by the names and addresses of all stockholders owning or holding 1 percent or more of the total amount of stock. If not owned by a corporation, give the names and addresses of the individual owners. If owned by a partnership or other unincorporated firm, give its name and address as well as those of each individual owner. If the publication is published by a nonprofit organization, give its name and address.)

Full Name	Complete Mailing Address
WHOLLY OWNED SUBSIDIARY OF REED/ELSEVIER, US HOLDINGS	1600 JOHN F KENNEDY BLVD. SUITE 1800 PHILADELPHIA, PA, 19103-2899

11. Known Bondholders, Mortgagees, and Other Security Holders Owning or Holding 1 Percent or More of Total Amount of Bonds, Mortgages, or Other Securities. If none, check box ► ☐ None

Full Name	Complete Mailing Address
N/A	

12. Tax Status (For completion by nonprofit organizations authorized to mail at nonprofit rates) (Check one)
The purpose, function, and nonprofit status of this organization and the exempt status for federal income tax purposes:
☒ Has Not Changed During Preceding 12 Months
☐ Has Changed During Preceding 12 Months (Publisher must submit explanation of change with this statement)

PS Form 3526, July 2014 [Page 1 of 4 (see instructions page 4)] PSN: 7530-01-000-9931 PRIVACY NOTICE: See our privacy policy on www.usps.com.

---

13. Publication Title	14. Issue Date for Circulation Data Below
DENTAL CLINICS OF NORTH AMERICA	JULY 2019

15. Extent and Nature of Circulation			Average No. Copies Each Issue During Preceding 12 Months	No. Copies of Single Issue Published Nearest to Filing Date
a. Total Number of Copies (Net press run)			243	281
b. Paid Circulation (By Mail and Outside the Mail)	(1)	Mailed Outside-County Paid Subscriptions Stated on PS Form 3541 (Include paid distribution above nominal rate, advertiser's proof copies, and exchange copies)	119	146
	(2)	Mailed In-County Paid Subscriptions Stated on PS Form 3541 (Include paid distribution above nominal rate, advertiser's proof copies, and exchange copies)	0	0
	(3)	Paid Distribution Outside the Mails Including Sales Through Dealers and Carriers, Street Vendors, Counter Sales, and Other Paid Distribution Outside USPS®	82	106
	(4)	Paid Distribution by Other Classes of Mail Through the USPS (e.g. First-Class Mail®)	0	0
c. Total Paid Distribution [Sum of 15b (1), (2), (3), and (4)]		►	201	252
d. Free or Nominal Rate Distribution (By Mail and Outside the Mail)	(1)	Free or Nominal Rate Outside-County Copies included on PS Form 3541	32	16
	(2)	Free or Nominal Rate In-County Copies Included on PS Form 3541	0	0
	(3)	Free or Nominal Rate Copies Mailed at Other Classes Through the USPS (e.g. First-Class Mail)	0	0
	(4)	Free or Nominal Rate Distribution Outside the Mail (Carriers or other means)	32	16
e. Total Free or Nominal Rate Distribution (Sum of 15d (1), (2), (3) and (4))		►	233	268
f. Total Distribution (Sum of 15c and 15e)		►	10	13
g. Copies not Distributed (See Instructions to Publishers #4 (page #3))		►	243	281
h. Total (Sum of 15f and g)			86.27%	94.03%
i. Percent Paid (15c divided by 15f times 100)		►		

* If you are claiming electronic copies, go to line 16 on page 3. If you are not claiming electronic copies, skip to line 17 on page 3.

16. Electronic Copy Circulation		Average No. Copies Each Issue During Preceding 12 Months	No. Copies of Single Issue Published Nearest to Filing Date
a. Paid Electronic Copies	►		
b. Total Paid Print Copies (Line 15c) + Paid Electronic Copies (Line 16a)	►		
c. Total Print Distribution (Line 15f) + Paid Electronic Copies (Line 16a)	►		
d. Percent Paid (Both Print & Electronic Copies) (16b divided by 16c × 100)	►		

☒ I certify that 50% of all my distributed copies (electronic and print) are paid above a nominal price.

17. Publication of Statement of Ownership
☒ If the publication is a general publication, publication of this statement is required. Will be printed ☐ Publication not required.
in the OCTOBER 2019 issue of this publication.

18. Signature and Title of Editor, Publisher, Business Manager, or Owner

STEPHEN R. BUSHING - INVENTORY DISTRIBUTION CONTROL MANAGER

Stephen R. Bushing Date 9/18/2019

I certify that all information furnished on this form is true and complete. I understand that anyone who furnishes false or misleading information on this form or who omits material or information requested on the form may be subject to criminal sanctions (including fines and imprisonment) and/or civil sanctions (including civil penalties).

PS Form 3526, July 2014 (Page 2 of 4)   PRIVACY NOTICE: See our privacy policy on www.usps.com

Moving?

Make sure your subscription moves with you!

To notify us of your new address, find your **Clinics Account Number** (located on your mailing label above your name), and contact customer service at:

Email: journalscustomerservice-usa@elsevier.com

800-654-2452 (subscribers in the U.S. & Canada)
314-447-8871 (subscribers outside of the U.S. & Canada)

Fax number: 314-447-8029

Elsevier Health Sciences Division
Subscription Customer Service
3251 Riverport Lane
Maryland Heights, MO 63043

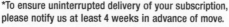
*To ensure uninterrupted delivery of your subscription,
please notify us at least 4 weeks in advance of move.

Printed and bound by CPI Group (UK) Ltd, Croydon, CR0 4YY

03/10/2024

01040479-0016